T0226502

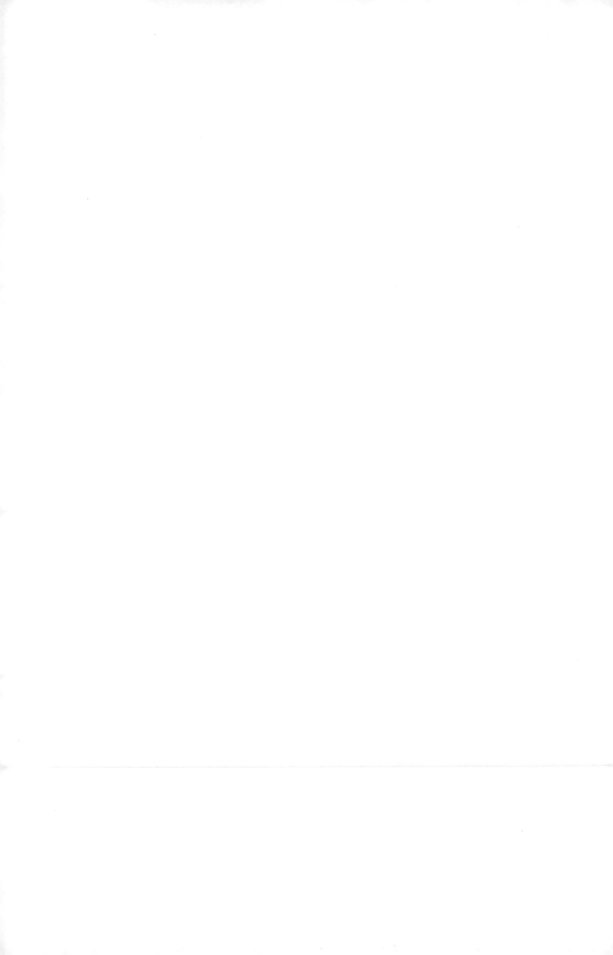

His Bundle Pacing

Editors

PRAMOD DESHMUKH
KENNETH A. ELLENBOGEN

CARDIAC ELECTROPHYSIOLOGY CLINICS

Consulting Editors
RANJAN K. THAKUR
ANDREA NATALE

September 2018 • Volume 10 • Number 3

ELSEVIER

1600 John F. Kennedy Boulevard • Suite 1800 • Philadelphia, Pennsylvania, 19103-2899

http://www.theclinics.com

CARDIAC ELECTROPHYSIOLOGY CLINICS Volume 10, Number 3
September 2018 ISSN 1877-9182, ISBN-13: 978-0-323-64221-7

Editor: Stacy Eastman
Developmental Editor: Donald Mumford

Cardiac Electrophysiology Clinics (ISSN 1877-9182) is published quarterly by Elsevier Inc., 360 Park Avenue South, New York, NY 10010-1710. Months of issue are March, June, September, and December. Subscription prices are $215.00 per year for US individuals, $344.00 per year for US institutions, $236.00 per year for Canadian individuals, $415.00 per year for Canadian institutions, $299.00 per year for international individuals, $415.00 per year for international institutions and $100.00 per year for US, Canadian and international students/residents. To receive student/resident rate, orders must be accompanied by name of affilliated institution, date of term, and the signature of program/residency coordinator on institution letterhead. Orders will be billed at individual rate until proof of status is received. Foreign air speed delivery is included in all Clinics subscription prices. All prices are subject to change without notice. **POSTMASTER:** Send address changes to Cardiac Electrophysiology Clinics, Elsevier Health Sciences Division, Subscription Customer Service, 3251 Riverport Lane, Maryland Heights, MO 63043. **Customer Service: 1-800-654-2452 (US and Canada). From outside of the US and Canada, call 314-477-8871. Fax: 314-447-8029. E-mail: JournalsCustomerService-usa@elsevier.com (for print support); JournalsOnlineSupport-usa@elsevier.com (for online support).**

Reprints. For copies of 100 or more of articles in this publication, please contact the Commercial Reprints Department, Elsevier Inc., 360 Park Avenue South, New York, NY 10010-1710. Tel.: 212-633-3874; Fax: 212-633-3820; E-mail: reprints@elsevier.com.

Cardiac Electrophysiology Clinics is covered in *MEDLINE/PubMed (Index Medicus).*

Contributors

CONSULTING EDITORS

RANJAN K. THAKUR, MD, MPH, MBA, FHRS
Professor of Medicine and Director, Arrhythmia
Service, Thoracic and Cardiovascular Institute,
Sparrow Health System, Michigan State
University, Lansing, Michigan, USA

ANDREA NATALE, MD, FACC, FHRS
Executive Medical Director, Texas
Cardiac Arrhythmia Institute, St. David's
Medical Center, Austin, Texas, USA;
Consulting Professor, Division of Cardiology,
Stanford University, Palo Alto, California, USA;
Adjunct Professor of Medicine, Heart and
Vascular Center, Case Western Reserve
University, Cleveland, Ohio, USA; Director,
Interventional Electrophysiology, Scripps
Clinic, San Diego, California, USA; Senior
Clinical Director, EP Services, California
Pacific Medical Center, San Francisco,
California, USA

EDITORS

PRAMOD DESHMUKH, MD
Director of Electrophysiology Services, Guthrie
Health Care System, Sayre, Pennsylvania, USA

KENNETH A. ELLENBOGEN, MD
Division of Cardiovascular Diseases, Virginia
Commonwealth University Health Science
Center, VCU School of Medicine, Medical
College of Virginia Hospitals, Richmond,
Virginia, USA

AUTHORS

SAMUEL J. ASIRVATHAM, MD
Professor of Medicine and Pediatrics,
Division of Heart Rhythm, Department of
Cardiovascular Diseases, Mayo Clinic,
Rochester, Minnesota, USA

SUBIR BHATIA, MD
Division of Internal Medicine, Department of
Medicine, Mayo Clinic, Rochester, Minnesota,
USA

JAMES D. CHANG, MD
Department of Medicine, Cardiovascular
Division, Beth Israel Deaconess Medical
Center, Harvard Medical School, Boston,
Massachusetts, USA

GOPI DANDAMUDI, MD, FHRS
System Medical Director, Indiana University
Health Cardiac Electrophysiology Program
Director, Indiana University Health Atrial
Fibrillation Center, Assistant Professor of
Medicine, Indiana University School of
Medicine, Indiana, USA

AMRISH DESHMUKH, MD
Chief Resident, Department of Medicine,
The University of Chicago, Chicago, Illinois,
USA

PRAMOD DESHMUKH, MD
Director of Electrophysiology Services,
Guthrie Health Care System, Sayre,
Pennsylvania, USA

SUBODH DEVABHAKTUNI, MD
Indiana University School of Medicine,
Indianapolis, Indiana, USA

ELISA EBRILLE, MD
Department of Medicine, Cardiovascular
Division, Beth Israel Deaconess Medical
Center, Harvard Medical School, Boston,
Massachusetts, USA

KENNETH A. ELLENBOGEN, MD
Division of Cardiovascular Diseases, Virginia
Commonwealth University Health Science
Center, VCU School of Medicine, Medical
College of Virginia Hospitals, Richmond,
Virginia, USA

WEIJIAN HUANG, MD, FHRS
Department of Cardiology, The First Affiliated
Hospital of Wenzhou Medical University, Key
Lab of Cardiovascular Disease of Wenzhou,
Wenzhou, China

JAYANTHI N. KONERU, MBBS
Associate Professor of Medicine
(Cardiology),Fellowship Program Director,
Division of Cardiology, VCU School of
Medicine, Richmond, Virginia, USA

UGUR KUCUK, MD
Division of Heart Rhythm, Department of
Cardiovascular Diseases, Mayo Clinic,
Rochester, Minnesota, USA

UMASHANKAR LAKSHMANADOSS, MD
Cardiac Electrophysiologist, Cardiac
Electrophysiology Division, Ballad Health
CVA Heart Institute, Kingsport, Tennessee,
USA

DANIEL L. LUSTGARTEN, MD, PhD, FHRS
Professor of Medicine, The University of
Vermont College of Medicine, The University of
Vermont Medical Center, Burlington, Vermont,
USA

PHILIP L. MAR, MD
Indiana University School of Medicine,
Indianapolis, Indiana, USA

FAISAL M. MERCHANT, MD
Cardiology Division, Emory University School
of Medicine, Atlanta, Georgia, USA

SUNEET MITTAL, MD
Valley Health System and The Snyder Center
for Comprehensive Atrial Fibrillation,
Ridgewood, New Jersey, USA

SIVA K. MULPURU, MD
Division of Heart Rhythm, Department of
Cardiovascular Diseases, Mayo Clinic,
Rochester, Minnesota, USA

HARSIMRAN SAINI, MD, PhD
VCU School of Medicine, Medical College
of Virginia Hospitals, Richmond, Virginia,
USA

BENJAMIN J. SCHERLAG, PhD
Department of Medicine, Heart Rhythm
Institute of Oklahoma, The University of
Oklahoma Health Sciences Center, Oklahoma
City, Oklahoma, USA

**PARIKSHIT S. SHARMA, MD, MPH, FACC,
FHRS**
Assistant Professor, Division of Cardiology,
Rush University Medical Center, Chicago,
Illinois, USA

JONATHAN SHIRAZI, MD
Indiana University School of Medicine,
Indianapolis, Indiana, USA

LAN SU, MD
Department of Cardiology, The First Affiliated
Hospital of Wenzhou Medical University, Key
Lab of Cardiovascular Disease of Wenzhou,
Wenzhou, China

FAIZ A. SUBZPOSH, MD
Geisinger Heart Institute, Wilkes-Barre,
Pennsylvania, USA

ALAN SUGRUE, MBChB
Division of Heart Rhythm, Department of
Cardiovascular Diseases, Mayo Clinic,
Rochester, Minnesota, USA

RICHARD TROHMAN, MD, MBA
Professor, Division of Cardiology, Rush
University Medical Center, Chicago, Illinois,
USA

RODERICK TUNG, MD
Associate Professor of Medicine, Director
of Electrophysiology, Center for Arrhythmia
Care, Pritzker School of Medicine, The
University of Chicago Medicine, Chicago,
Illinois, USA

GAURAV A. UPADHYAY, MD
Assistant Professor of Medicine, Center for
Arrhythmia Care, Pritzker School of Medicine,
The University of Chicago Medicine, Chicago,
Illinois, USA

VAIBHAV R. VAIDYA, MBBS
Division of Heart Rhythm, Department
of Cardiovascular Diseases, Mayo Clinic,
Rochester, Minnesota, USA

PUGAZHENDHI VIJAYARAMAN, MD, FHRS
Director, Cardiac Electrophysiology, Geisinger
Heart Institute, Wilkes-Barre, Pennsylvania,
USA; Fellowship Director, Cardiac
Electrophysiology, Geisinger Medical Center,
Danville, Pennsylvania, USA; Associate
Professor of Medicine, Geisinger
Commonwealth School of Medicine, Scranton,
Pennsylvania, USA

SHENGJIE WU, MD
Department of Cardiology, The First Affiliated
Hospital of Wenzhou Medical University, Key
Lab of Cardiovascular Disease of Wenzhou,
Wenzhou, China

PETER J. ZIMETBAUM, MD
Department of Medicine, Cardiovascular
Division, Beth Israel Deaconess Medical
Center, Harvard Medical School, Boston,
Massachusetts, USA

Contents

> One of the drawbacks of permanent His bundle pacing has been the relatively high pacing thresholds. The present experimental study was proposed to address this issue. In this article the authors present preliminary evidence that His bundle pacing can be achieved with subthreshold stimulation, thereby providing for increased battery life and consequently longer replacement intervals. Possible mechanisms underlying the paradoxical effects of subthreshold stimulation before and after the onset of complete atrioventricular block are also discussed.

> Pacing-induced cardiomyopathy (PICM) is a well-described phenomenon that occurs in a minority of patients exposed to high-burden right ventricular (RV) pacing. Although several risk factors may identify patients at increased risk of PICM, many individuals tolerate high-burden RV pacing for many years without obviously deleterious effects, and the ability to identify those at highest risk remains insufficient. Treatment of PICM has primarily involved upgrade to cardiac resynchronization therapy once signs of cardiomyopathy manifest. The emergence of His bundle pacing may offer an opportunity to prevent PICM before it occurs.

> Tricuspid regurgitation is increasingly recognized as a clinically significant valvular condition. The role of multiple pacemaker and implantable cardiac defibrillator leads in distortion of the valve structure and the risk of trauma to the valve and subvalvular apparatus with lead extraction contribute to the development of tricuspid regurgitation (TR). There is a clinical imperative to better understand the optimal way to diagnose lead-related TR, risk factors for the development of TR, and optimal strategies to mitigate this problem.

> This article summarizes the initial experience with permanent His bundle pacing, the lessons learned, and the concepts that have been developed in the subsequent decade of experience with His bundle pacing. This article also addresses the

advancements in technology, which have allowed His bundle pacing to be more widely adopted and used in various clinical situations.

His Bundle (Conduction System) Pacing: A Contemporary Appraisal

Alan Sugrue, Subir Bhatia, Vaibhav R. Vaidya, Ugur Kucuk, Siva K. Mulpuru, and Samuel J. Asirvatham

The His bundle (conduction system) is an attractive target for physiologic pacing because it uses the native conduction system. Although the potential benefits of conduction system pacing were recognized in the 1970s, in the past 2 decades, it has grown in interest as a potentially preferred method of ventricular stimulation in appropriate patients. This article provides an appraisal of conduction system pacing, with focus on anatomy, physiology, tools, and techniques, as well as an appraisal of current published data and thoughts on future directions.

An Electro-Anatomic Atlas of His Bundle Pacing: Combining Fluoroscopic Imaging and Recorded Electrograms

Parikshit S. Sharma and Richard Trohman

Permanent His bundle pacing (PHBP) has gained significant popularity given improved implant success rates given better tools and increasing data on the clinical benefits of PHBP. In this article, the authors review the relevant anatomy of the bundle of His and help correlate PHBP implant characteristics with patient anatomy using fluoroscopic and electroanatomic correlations.

His Bundle Pacing: Getting on the Learning Curve

Daniel L. Lustgarten

Permanent His bundle pacing prevents ventricular dyssynchrony in patients who depend on ventricular pacing and can provide an alternative means to implementing cardiac resynchronization therapy in patients with bundle branch disease and congestive heart failure. Adoption of His bundle pacing, however, has lagged in part owing to perceived and real challenges in performing the procedure well and durably. This article focuses on what is required to get on the learning curve and developing technical competence.

How to Perform His Bundle Pacing: Tools and Techniques

Subodh Devabhaktuni, Philip L. Mar, Jonathan Shirazi, and Gopi Dandamudi

Recently, permanent His bundle pacing (HBP) has emerged as a viable pacing strategy for chronic ventricular pacing. It allows for recruitment of the native His-Purkinje system thereby preventing pacing-induced ventricular dyssynchrony seen in traditional right ventricular pacing. Current tools allow for relatively good success rates for implantation. Understanding the various responses to HBP is crucial for long-term success. With better tools and unique pacing and sensing algorithms designed specifically for this form of pacing, HBP is likely to increase as a tool for long-term pacing therapy.

Hemodynamics of His Bundle Pacing

Amrish Deshmukh, Umashankar Lakshmanadoss, and Pramod Deshmukh

In addition to the His bundle, numerous other sites have been evaluated as more physiologic alternatives to pacing at the right ventricular apex. Several hemodynamic studies have shown the benefit of His bundle pacing and septal pacing in comparison with right ventricular apical pacing. This article summarizes this literature and presents hemodynamic data in an intrapatient study examining His bundle pacing, right ventricular septal pacing, and right ventricular apical pacing.

CARDIAC ELECTROPHYSIOLOGY CLINICS

THE CLINICS ARE AVAILABLE ONLINE!
Access your subscription at:
www.theclinics.com

Dedication

Every advance in science is based on previous knowledge, and this text is no exception. On a personal level, I had the good fortune to be taught by Professor Dabholkar. In addition to imparting a sound foundation in human physiology, he fostered my spirit of scientific inquiry. Finally, Swami Dayananda Saraswati, a master teacher of Vedanta, taught me self inquiry and inspired an invaluable clarity of mind and spirit.

I dedicate my efforts to both of them.

Pramod Deshmukh, MD
Director, Arrhythmia Service
Guthrie Health Care System
1 Guthrie Square
Sayre, PA 18840, USA

E-mail address:
prmode@yahoo.com

Card Electrophysiol Clin 10 (2018) xi
https://doi.org/10.1016/j.ccep.2018.07.002
1877-9182/18/© 2018 Elsevier Inc. All rights reserved.

Foreword
His Bundle Pacing: A 100-Year Journey

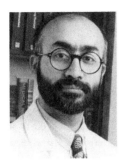 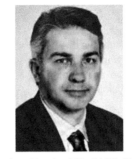

Ranjan K. Thakur, MD, MPH, MBA, FHRS   Andrea Natale, MD, FACC, FHRS

Consulting Editors

We welcome readers to the current issue of *Cardiac Electrophysiology Clinics* on His bundle pacing. Like many other fields in medicine, the story of His bundle pacing is quite interesting, demonstrating the value of physiological discoveries long forgotten and grit and determination of a lone ranger to champion an idea.

Wiggers[1] had shown the deleterious hemodynamic effects of ventricular pacing almost 100 years ago. However, when cardiac pacing developed in the 1960s, endocardial ventricular pacing was an obvious way forward. Unfortunately, it took us more than four decades to realize that right ventricular pacing may be harmful, and biventricular pacing was adopted as a method to mitigate the harm.

Dr Deshmukh's contribution to the field of His bundle pacing is to be lauded. Before pacing-induced cardiomyopathy became well appreciated in electrophysiology circles, spurred by the work of Wiggers, the teachings of his own physiology professor in medical school, and the animal work by Dr Scherlag, Dr Deshmukh embarked on clinical His bundle pacing to achieve physiologic ventricular activation more than twenty years ago. The magnitude of this challenge was enormous because there were no special tools available. He used commercially available active-fixation leads and manually formed stylets to direct the tip of the pacing lead to the His-bundle. An average implant lasted several hours; yet he persisted and his seminal work was published almost two decades ago.[2] While demonstrating the feasibility of His bundle pacing resulting in synchronous ventricular activation and hemodynamic benefits, Dr Deshmukh also added to the established criteria for demonstrating selective His bundle pacing. He singularly transformed an idea into clinical reality.

Since his initial publication in 2000, although adopted slowly, the benefit of His bundle pacing has sparked the imagination of electrophysiologists, and some investigators have made valuable contributions and demonstrated its utility in various circumstances. However, until recently, His bundle pacing was the purview of a few interested electrophysiologists. Recently, there has been an upsurge in interest and widespread diffusion of this technique, evidenced by an increasing number of laboratories starting to use it.

This issue of *Cardiac Electrophysiology Clinics* focuses on the current utility of His bundle pacing, its uses under various conditions, advantages, and challenges. Going forward, we see His bundle pacing as a preferred site for pacing, whenever it

Card Electrophysiol Clin 10 (2018) xiii–xiv
https://doi.org/10.1016/j.ccep.2018.07.003
1877-9182/18/© 2018 Published by Elsevier Inc.

can be achieved. But, a lot more needs to be learned yet, and we need better leads and delivery mechanisms to help accomplish it quickly and more reliably. To reach that goal, we will need help and innovation from our colleagues in the pacing industry.

We want to thank Dr Deshmukh and Dr Ellenbogen for editing an excellent issue of *Cardiac Electrophysiology Clinics*. Many of the contributors are established investigators in the field, and we thank them for their excellent articles. We hope that the readers will find this issue informative and useful in their own journey to delivering physiologic pacing via the His bundle.

Ranjan K. Thakur, MD, MPH, MBA, FHRS
Sparrow Thoracic and Cardiovascular Institute
Michigan State University
1440 East Michigan Avenue, Suite 400
Lansing, MI 48912, USA

Andrea Natale, MD, FACC, FHRS
Texas Cardiac Arrhythmia Institute
Center for Atrial Fibrillation at
St. David's Medical Center
1015 East 32nd Street, Suite 516
Austin, TX 78705, USA

E-mail addresses:
thakur@msu.edu (R.K. Thakur)
andrea.natale@stdavids.com (A. Natale)

REFERENCES

1. Wiggers CJ. The muscular reactions of mammalian ventricles to artificial surface stimuli. Am J Physiol 1925;73:346–78.
2. Deshmukh P, Casavant DA, Romanyshan M, et al. Permanent, direct His-bundle pacing. Circulation 2000;101:869–77.

Preface
His Bundle Pacing: Everything Old Is New Again

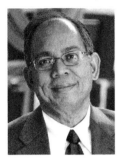   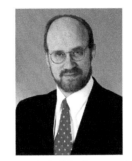

Pramod Deshmukh, MD   Kenneth A. Ellenbogen, MD

Editors

The development of His bundle pacing is both a story of technological advancement and a return to old physiologic principles. Electrical pacing of the heart began as an open-chest procedure performed by surgeons. It was only with the advent of the transvenous approach that cardiologists began to implant pacemakers. Subsequent developments then focused on improvements in technology with advancements in batteries, digital electronics, programming functions, and leads. During this time, the seminal work of Dr Wiggers from 1925, which identified the deleterious impact of ventricular pacing, appeared to be forgotten and pacing in the ventricular musculature remained the standard.

Reflecting on our early experience, I feel very lucky to be trained as an electrophysiologist prior to implanting pacemakers. Thanks to this background, an excellent physiology teacher, and perhaps the naiveté of an early operator, we first performed selective His bundle pacing with a desire to maintain normal ventricular activation. After establishing it was indeed possible, the challenges early on made it important to define selective His pacing. In addition to published criteria by Dr Sherlag, the third criteria (all-or-none) was defined and added. This third criterion is now labeled "single capture threshold" and forms the basis of select versus nonselect pacing.

Since this initial experience, His bundle pacing has proliferated and has been employed in diverse settings. The contributors to this issue deserve special praise for reproducing our observations with systematic study and then carrying them much further into new contexts. It is especially notable that the field of His bundle pacing has been driven primarily by clinicians seeking to best treat their patients rather than by funding from the medical industry. It is through their vigorous enthusiasm that His bundle pacing has become widespread, and there is now the development of specialized tools for its performance.

This text seeks to summarize the physiology of His bundle pacing, practical knowledge useful in its adoption, and the growing wealth of experience of utilizing His bundle pacing in various contexts. We hope that in its readings others will continue to adopt His bundle pacing into their practice and be inspired to join in advancing the field.

There are many people without whom this issue would not be complete. I would like to thank my medical school professor, Dr Dabholkar, for giving me a solid foundation in physiology. Personal encouragement by Dr Sherlag and the kind review by Dr Scheinman were also of immense help in the early days. I would like to thank Ken for his

Card Electrophysiol Clin 10 (2018) xv–xvi
https://doi.org/10.1016/j.ccep.2018.07.001
1877-9182/18/© 2018 Published by Elsevier Inc.

insights, contributions, and guidance for this issue. Last but not least, the contributors to this issue deserve a special thank you, as without their efforts it would not be published.

Pramod Deshmukh, MD
Director, Arrhythmia Service
Guthrie Health Care System
1 Guthrie Square
Sayre, PA 18840, USA

Kenneth A. Ellenbogen, MD
Division of Cardiovascular Diseases
Virginia Commonwealth University
Health Science Center
1200 East Marshall Street
Gateway Building, 3rd Floor, 3-216
Richmond, VA 23298, USA

E-mail addresses:
prmode@yahoo.com (P. Deshmukh)
ken.ellenbogen@gmail.com (K.A. Ellenbogen)

Subthreshold Stimulation for His Bundle Pacing

Benjamin J. Scherlag, PhD

KEYWORDS

- Direct current • Long- and short-duration • Atrioventricular • His bundle pacing
- Sub-threshold stimulation • Atrioventricular block

KEY POINTS

- The delivery of long- or short-duration direct current stimuli to the His bundle at an intensity just below the threshold to induce excitation in the early stages of ischemia at the His bundle induced complete atrioventricular (AV) block, whereas when complete AV block occurred these subthreshold stimuli restored 1:1 AV conduction.
- Subthreshold stimulation should reduce the high thresholds levels presently required for His bundle pacing and provide longer battery replacement intervals.

INTRODUCTION

Early experimental studies comparing synchronous A-His bundle and A-right ventricle (RV) apex pacing demonstrated a significantly greater response in regard to left ventricular pressure, rate of increase in left ventricular pressure, and aortic flow by His bundle pacing than RV apex pacing at any atrioventricular (AV) paced interval.[1] Within a decade later, 2 clinical studies showed that His bundle pacing could normalize the QRS in patients with various forms of bundle branch block.[2,3] These benefits of His bundle pacing could not be realized until the development of permanent His bundle pacing in 2000.[4] Using a screw-in lead at the His bundle, Deshmukh and colleagues were able to maintain long-term His bundle pacing in patients with cardiomyopathies, providing substantial improvement in ventricular function. Recently, permanent His bundle pacing has emerged as a routine clinical procedure for the treatment of patients with heart failure with associated AV block and bundle branch block electrocardiographic patterns.[5]

One of the major drawbacks that has been encountered with His bundle pacing has been the higher threshold needed to pace compared with RV apex pacing.[5] A consequence of the higher thresholds has been greater battery drain and shorter pulse generator replacement intervals. In this article, the author present preliminary evidence that His bundle pacing can be achieved with subthreshold stimulation, thereby providing for increased battery life and consequently longer replacement intervals.

METHODS

Adult mongrel dogs (n = 10) were anesthetized with sodium pentobarbital. Under controlled ventilation, the left side of the thorax was opened at the fourth intercostal space and the heart exposed by a pericardiotomy. The left atrial appendage was reflected, and the area of the bifurcation of the main left coronary artery was dissected in order to expose the anterior descending, anterior septal, and circumflex arteries. A silk ligature was looped around the anterior septal artery for later ligation of

Conflict of Interest: None declared.
Funding Source: Supported by an unrestricted grant from the Helen and Wilton Webster Foundation through the Oklahoma Research foundation MISCA COM083-COM09006.
The Department of Medicine, The Heart Rhythm Institute, The University of Oklahoma Health Sciences Center, 800 Stanton L. Young Boulevard, Suite 5400, Oklahoma City, OK 73104, USA
E-mail address: benjamin-scherlag@ouhsc.edu

Card Electrophysiol Clin 10 (2018) 431–435
https://doi.org/10.1016/j.ccep.2018.05.004

this vessel. An electrode catheter was inserted into a carotid artery and wedged at the aortic root for stable recording of the His bundle potential, which also allowed for stable His bundle pacing.[6] In order to reduce the heart rate, stimulation (0.5 msec duration, 20 Hz, 1–10V) of the vagosympathetic trunk was accomplished via 2 Teflon-coated silver wires inserted into the exposed portion of the right or left nerve trunk.[7] To increase the heart rate, stimuli from a Grass stimulator S-88 and stimulus isolation unit (SIU5) were delivered to the atrium at 150 to 330 beats/min via stainless steel wires inserted into the left atrial appendage.

Subthreshold stimulation to the His bundle electrode on the second channel of the stimulator. The duration and intensity of the second output could be independently adjusted.

In addition to the electrograms, 2 or more standard electrocardiographic leads were recorded; in most cases leads II and aVR were used. Electrograms were recorded using frequency limits between 40 and 200 Hz, whereas electrocardiographic leads were recorded using standard frequency limits between 0.1 and 200 Hz. All recordings were registered on an oscilloscopic, photographic recorder at paper speeds between 25 and 200 mm/s. A peripheral vein was cannulated for administration of drugs and a peripheral artery was also cannulated for monitoring blood pressure by standard techniques.

Definition of Terms

The diagnosis of right and left bundle branch block was made from the electrocardiographic patterns in leads II and aVR. Normally in the dog, lead II inscribes a QR or QRS configuration with a QRS duration of 41 ± 8 msec, whereas lead aVR has an rS or rSr' pattern.[8] Right bundle branch block results in a marked decrease of the amplitude of the R wave in lead II and the S wave in lead aVR, with the development of a terminal broad frequently slurred S wave in lead II and an R wave in lead aVR. Lesser degrees of right bundle branch block give rise to intermediate changes. Right bundle branch block does not usually alter the initial QRS vectors. The QRS duration during complete bundle branch block usually increases to greater than 80 ± 10 msec.[8]

RESULTS

Before ligation of the anterior septal artery, recordings were made during atrial pacing at rates up to 300 beats/min. All animals showed Wenckebach type block localized at proximal recording site of the His bundle deflection at rates between 270 and 300 beats/min. After one-stage ligation of the anterior septal artery, vagal slowing of the heart

rate was used to prevent or mitigate serious ventricular arrhythmias that were seen during the first 20 min after arterial ligation.[9–11] During this period, 2 of the 10 animals developed ventricular fibrillation and were lost from the study. The other 8 were followed for at least 2 hours until complete heart block developed. When the arrhythmic period passed (15–25 min), the heart rate was increased by atrial pacing up to 270 to 300 beats/min, just below the rate that AV nodal block occurred, in order to exacerbate the development of ischemic injury in the His bundle and the proximal bundle branches.[9,10]

In the control state, before anterior septal artery ligation, a long-duration constant current stimulus whose intensity (5 mA) was just below that which induced activation of the His bundle at the stimulus onset (make shock) or at the offset (break shock) did not result in His bundle activation (**Fig. 1**, top panel).

Thirty minutes after septal artery ligation, the same-intensity long-duration stimulus resulted in complete AV block with an idioventricular escape beat. Note that before and after the application of the long-duration pulse, the electrocardiogram indicated that ischemic injury to the His-Purkinje system resulted in the development of incomplete right bundle branch block (see **Fig. 1**, middle panel).

After 2 hours, when complete heart block was recorded with a slow idioventricular rhythm, the same long-duration pulse (5 mA) restored 1:1 AV conduction showing a right bundle block pattern. Note that the break shock just after atrial activation caused premature His bundle excitation with a shortened P-R interval. Cessation of the long-duration pulse was followed by resumption of AV heart block (see **Fig. 1**, bottom panel).

Another method for achieving these results using subthreshold stimulation was the coupling of atrial pacing at 180/min from channel one of the S88 stimulator to a second channel whose output was delivered to the His bundle (see Methods). **Fig. 2** shows atrial pacing, started during complete heart block (top panel), coupled with a short-duration (15 ms) constant current stimulus (5 mA) delivered to the His bundle 70 msec after each atrial pacing stimulus. Note the restoration of 1:1 conduction with an incomplete right bundle branch block pattern (middle panel). A slight reduction (4 mA) of the stimuli delivered to the His bundle resulted in 2:1 conduction with maintenance of incomplete right bundle branch block (bottom panel).

DISCUSSION
Major Findings

The delivery of long- or short-duration stimuli at an intensity just below the threshold to induce

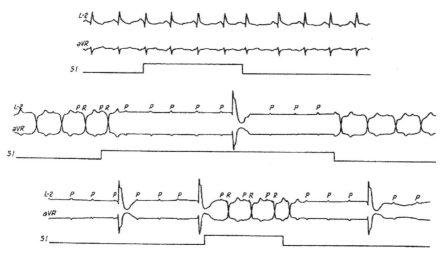

Fig. 1. Electrocardiogram leads 2 and aVR were recorded. Long-duration direct current (DC) pulses applied to the His bundle during the course of acute ischemia of the atrioventricular (AV) junction. (*Top panel*) At baseline, before ischemia induced by ligation of the anterior septal artery, a long-duration subthreshold DC pulse (5 mA) applied to the His bundle shows no response. (*Middle panel*) Thirty to sixty minutes after induced ischemia, incomplete right bundle branch block was recorded; the same-intensity (5 mA) DC pulse applied to the His bundle induced complete heart block with a ventricular escape beat. (*Lower panel*) Two hours of AV junctional ischemia resulted in complete heart block with a slow idioventricular escape rhythm. A DC pulse (5 mA) restores 1: 1 AV conduction with incomplete right bundle branch block.

excitation during 2 hours of ischemic damage to the His bundle area after anterior septal artery ligation in the canine and affected AV conduction: these subthreshold stimuli in the early stages of ischemia induced complete AV block, whereas when complete AV block occurred these subthreshold stimuli restored 1:1 AV conduction.

Background

In previous reports, the authors demonstrated that conduction disorders occurred in the dog heart in the interval between 30 minutes and 2 hours after anterior septal artery ligation. Ischemic damage to the His bundle and proximal bundle branch could be exacerbated by high-rate atrial pacing.[9–11] It could be argued that the use of subthreshold His bundle pacing to unmask susceptibility to heart block is restricted to situations involving ischemic insults to the area of the AV junction as in inferior myocardial infarction or when the main left coronary is compromised. However, an experimental study, in which peripheral myocardial ischemia induced by narrowing or ligation of the left anterior coronary artery was followed by block distal to the His bundle caused by either rapid atrial pacing or closely coupled premature atrial beats.[12]

Both experimental and clinical studies have reported that suprathreshold premature beats[12–14] or rapid atrial pacing[15] can induce AV block.

On the other hand, premature beats delivered during specific intervals within the cardiac cycle have been shown to restore 1:1 AV conduction.[14,16]

Mechanism of Action of Subthreshold Stimuli

The question arises as to what mechanism explains the observation that subthreshold stimuli, either long or short duration, applied in the early stages of the ischemically damaged His bundle can induce AV block; whereas, at a later stage, during stable AV block, the same subthreshold stimuli restores AV conduction. An earlier in vitro study[17] of the acutely damaged His bundle showed decreased action potential upstroke and some decrease in resting potential that was associated with various forms of bundle branch and AV block. At this acute stage the blocks were reversible. In contrast when complete AV block occurred, subthreshold stimuli delivered to the depolarized His bundle cells would cause hyperpolarization leading to restoration of AV conduction; however, the persistence of incomplete bundle branch block indicates that ischemic damage was not entirely reversed (see **Fig. 2**, middle panel).

Clinical Implications

The acute application of subthreshold stimulation to the His bundle to induce AV blocks could be tested in patients with implanted His bundle leads who have shown improvement in their cardiomyopathy with normal QRS durations.[4] On the

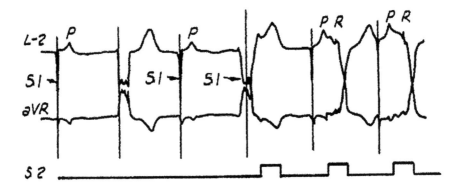

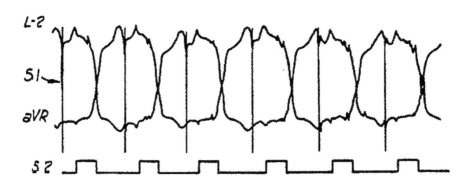

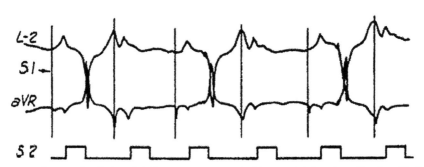

Fig. 2. Electrocardiogram leads 2 and aVR traces are separated by an atrial pacing stimulus, S1. A coupled short-duration DC pulse, S2 (5 mA) was delivered to the His bundle after each atrial paced beat. (*Top panel*) During the first 2 beats of AV heart block atrial pacing and coupled subthreshold stimulus, S1-S2 restored AV conduction (*Middle panel*) with incomplete right bundle branch block patterns. (*Lower panel*) Reducing S2 from 5 to 4 mA results in 2:1 AV block.

other hand, subthreshold pacing applied to the His bundle could be tested in patients in whom His bundle pacing has shown normalization of bundle branch block.[18] Would subthreshold pacing acutely, similarly reverse the bundle branch block pattern or some instances of complete heart block?

SUMMARY

The delivery of long- or short-duration direct current stimuli to the His bundle at an intensity just below the threshold to induce excitation in the early stages of ischemia at the His bundle induced complete AV block, whereas when complete AV block occurred these subthreshold stimuli restored 1:1 AV conduction.

REFERENCES

1. Kosowsky BD, Scherlag BJ, Damato AN. Reevaluation of the atrial contribution to ventricular function. Am J Cardiol 1968;21:518–24.
2. Narula OS. Longitudinal dissociation in the His bundle. Bundle branch block due to asynchronous conduction within the His bundle in man. Circulation 1977;56:996–1006.
3. El-Sherif N, Amat-Y-Leon F, Schonfeld C, et al. Normalization of bundle branch block patterns by distalHis bundle pacing. Clinical and experimental evidence of longitudinal dissociation in the pathologic His bundle. Circulation 1978;57:473–83.
4. Deshmukh P, Casavant D, Romanyshyn M, et al. Permanent direct His bundle pacing. A novel approach to cardiac pacing in patients with normal His-Purkinje activation. Circulation 2000;101:869–77.
5. Dandamudi G, Vijayaraman P. How to perform permanent His bundle pacing in routine clinical practice. Heart Rhythm 2016;13:1362–6.
6. Scherlag BJ, Abelleira JL, Samet P. Electrode catheter recordings from the His bundle and left bundle in the intact dog. In: Kao FF, Koizumi K, Vassale M, editors. Research in physiology. Bologna (Italy): Aulo Gaggi Editore; 1971. p. 223–31.
7. Lazzara R, Scherlag BJ, Robinson MJ, et al. Selective in situ parasympathetic control of the canine sino-atrial and atrioventricular node. Circ Res 1973;32:393–402.
8. Ettinger SJ, Sutter PF. Canine cardiology. Philadelphia: W B Saunders; 1970. p. 132–9.
9. Scherlag BJ, El-Sherif N, Lazzara R. Experimental model for the study of Mobitz II and paroxysmal atrioventricular block. Am J Cardiol 1974;34:309–17.
10. El-Sherif N, Scherlag BJ, Lazzara R. Conduction disorders in the canine proximal His-Purkinje system following acute myocardial ischemia. I. The pathophysiology of intra-His bundle block. Circulation 1974;49:847–57.
11. Lazzara R, El-Sherif N, Scherlag BJ. Disorders of cellular electrophysiology produced by ischemia of the canine His bundle. Circ Res 1975;36:444–54.
12. Scherlag BJ, Hope RR, Lazzara R. Proximal His-Purkinje conduction defects due to peripheral myocardial ischemia and infarction. Jpn Heart J 1979;20:495–510.
13. Coumel P, Fabiato A, Waynberger M, et al. Bradycardia-dependent atrio-ventricular block: Report of two cases of A-V block elicited by premature beats. J Electrocardiol 1971;4:168–77.
14. Rosenbaum MB, Elizari MV, Levi RJ, et al. Paroxysmal atrio-ventricular block related to hypopolarization and spontaneous diastolic depolarization. Chest 1973;63:678–88.
15. Dhingra RC, Wyndham C, Bauernfeind R, et al. Significance of block distal to the His bundle induced by atrial pacing in patients with chronic bifascicular block. Circulation 1979;60:1455–64.
16. Gonzalez MD, Scherlag BJ, Mabo P, et al. Conversion of Mobitz type II block to 1:1 conduction by premature ventricular beats. J Electrocardiol 1992; 25(suppl):165–72.
17. Scherlag BJ, El-Sherif N, Hope RR, et al. The significance of dissociation of conduction in the canine His bundle. Electrophysiological studies in vivo and in vitro. J Electrocardiol 1978;11:343–54.
18. Lustgarten DL, Calame S, Crespo EM, et al. Electrical resynchronization induced by direct His-bundle pacing. Heart Rhythm 2010;7:15–21.

Pacing-Induced Cardiomyopathy

Faisal M. Merchant, MD[a], Suneet Mittal, MD[b],*

KEYWORDS

- Pacing-induced cardiomyopathy • Pacemaker • High-burden right ventricular pacing

KEY POINTS

- Pacing-induced cardiomyopathy (PICM) is a well described phenomenon that occurs in a minority of patients exposed to high-burden right ventricular (RV) pacing.
- Although several risk factors may identify patients at increased risk of PICM, many individuals tolerate high-burden RV pacing for many years without obviously deleterious effects, and the ability to identify those at highest risk remains insufficient.
- Treatment of PICM has primarily involved upgrade to cardiac resynchronization therapy once signs of cardiomyopathy manifest.
- The emergence of His bundle pacing may offer an opportunity to prevent PICM before it occurs.

Over 1,000,000 pacemakers are implanted annually worldwide, with approximately half for a diagnosis of high-degree atrioventricular (AV) block.[1] Although many individuals tolerate high-burden right ventricle (RV) pacing for many years without clinically discernible adverse effects,[2] it has been increasingly recognized that chronic RV pacing may lead to compromised left ventricle (LV) function and may result in symptoms of heart failure (HF), a syndrome known as pacing-induced cardiomyopathy (PICM). Although the exact incidence of PICM and the risk factors that lead to its development continue to be defined, given the large number of pacemakers implanted and the significant percentage of patients with high-burden RV pacing, the potential public health and economic impacts of PICM are substantial, and strategies to prevent and treat it are of clinical importance.

INCIDENCE AND DEFINITIONS OF PACING-INDUCED CARDIOMYOPATHY

The reported incidence of PICM has varied based on different definitions used to identify the syndrome. The most commonly utilized definitions invoke a drop in LV ejection fraction (LVEF) in the setting of high-burden RV pacing. In a study of 257 patients with normal baseline LVEF, the incidence of PICM (defined as a drop in LVEF $\geq$10% and resulting in an LVEF <50%) was 19.5% at a mean follow-up of 3.3 years.[3] In a similar study, using a definition of drop in LVEF of greater than 5% from baseline in conjunction with symptoms of HF, in a cohort of 234 patients, Lee and colleagues[4] reported an incidence of PICM of 20.5% at a mean follow-up of 15.6 years. Using a broader definition of PICM to include both drop in LVEF (to $\leq$40%) or need for upgrade to cardiac resynchronization therapy (CRT), in a cohort of 823 patients with normal baseline LVEF (>50%) undergoing permanent pacemaker (PPM) implantation for complete heart block (CHB), Kiehl and colleagues[5] reported an incidence of PICM of 12.3% at a mean follow-up of 4.3 years. Among randomized, prospective data in the Pacing to Avoid Cardiac Enlargement (PACE) study, 177 patients with normal baseline LVEF were randomized to CRT pacing or RV pacing.[6] Although the

Disclosures: None (F.M. Merchant). Consultant to Abbott, Boston Scientific, and Medtronic (S. Mittal).
a Cardiology Division, Emory University School of Medicine, 550 Peachree Street North East, Atlanta, GA 3030, USA; b Valley Health System and The Snyder Center for Comprehensive Atrial Fibrillation, 223 North Van Dien Avenue, Ridgewood, NJ 07450, USA
* Corresponding author. 1 Linwood Avenue, Paramus, NJ 07652.
E-mail address: mittsu@valleyhealth.com

Card Electrophysiol Clin 10 (2018) 437–445
https://doi.org/10.1016/j.ccep.2018.05.005

inclusion criteria for the PACE study required LVEF greater than 45% at baseline, the mean LVEF of patients enrolled in the study was 61.7%. At 12 months, mean LVEF dropped to 54.8% in the RV pacing group, but remained stable at 62.2% in the CRT pacing cohort (P<.001). The decrement in LVEF in the RV pacing arm was also associated with a significant increase in LV systolic volume. During longer-term follow-up from the same study (mean 4.8 years), the groups continued to diverge, with further decrement in LVEF in the RV pacing group to a mean of 53.2% and continued increase in LV systolic volumes, whereas those parameters were stable in the CRT pacing arm.[7] Additionally, despite the relatively modest drop in LVEF in the RV pacing arm, the incidence of HF hospitalization in PACE was significantly greater in the RV pacing group (23.9 vs 14.6%, P = .006).

Although assessment of LVEF has featured prominently in many studies reporting the incidence of PICM, the development of HF symptoms or incidence of HF hospitalization also contributes importantly to the definition of the syndrome. In the MOde Selection Trial (MOST), comparing single-chamber ventricular pacing to dual-chamber pacing in sinus node dysfunction, in analyses adjusted for baseline covariates, the incidence of HF hospitalization was nearly 2.5 fold higher in the dual-chamber pacing arm among those with greater than 40% RV pacing burden compared with those with lower burdens of ventricular pacing.[8] In contrast to predominantly sinus node dysfunction in the MOST study, in a claims database of over 21,000 patients undergoing pacemaker implantation, the risk of a new HF diagnosis after device implant was significantly higher among those with a diagnosis of AV block (used as a surrogate for increased RV pacing burden), compared with those without a diagnosis of AV block (adjusted hazard ratio [HR] 1.62, 95% confidence interval [CI] 1.48 - 1.79).[9] Interestingly, in this analysis, the hazard associated with high-burden RV pacing was most notable within the first 6 months following pacemaker implantation, suggesting a more acute risk of HF symptoms than has been appreciated previously. Similarly, among patients with predominantly AV nodal disease in the Biventricular versus Right Ventricular Pacing in Heart Failure Patients with Atrioventricular Block (Block HF) study, the clinical composite score incorporating New York Heart Association (NYHA) class, HF hospitalization, and subjective assessment of HF symptoms and quality of life was significantly better in the CRT arm than among those randomized to RV only pacing.[10] Importantly, patients enrolled in Block HF already had some degree of LV dysfunction at baseline (LVEF <50%), and the results suggest that the hazard associated with high-burden RV pacing

may be even more notable among those with baseline impairment of LV function. In a cohort of patients with impaired LVEF who were candidates for defibrillator implantation, the Dual Chamber and VVI Implantable Defibrillator (DAVID) trial demonstrated that the cumulative incidence of death or HF hospitalization was over 30% at 18 months among those with greater than 40% RV pacing, compared with an incidence of less than 10% in the group with less than 40% RV pacing.[11] In a similar cohort of patients eligible for defibrillator implantation, the Multicenter Automatic Defibrillator Implantation Trial (MADIT) II demonstrated that at 3-year follow-up, RV pacing burden greater than 50% was associated with a nearly twofold increased risk of new or worsened HF, based on investigator-assessed symptoms or need for augmentation of pharmacologic therapy.[12]

In aggregate, these data suggest that approximately 10% to 20% of individuals with baseline normal LV function will develop a significant drop in LVEF within the first 3 to 4 years following high-burden RV pacing. For many of these patients, RV pacing also leads to the development of clinical HF symptoms and significantly increases the incidence of HF hospitalization. The risks associated with PICM may be even more notable among those with baseline impairments in LV function. Although a significant body of literature supports the existence of PICM as a distinct clinical syndrome, it appears likely that not all patients are equally susceptible to the detrimental effects of high-burden RV pacing. Among a cohort of 286 patients undergoing AV junction ablation resulting in obligate high-burden RV pacing, no significant decrement in LVEF was noted at a mean follow-up of 20 months, and the 10-year incidence of HF hospitalization in this cohort was only 8%.[2] In a similar single-center study from Germany, among 791 patients with baseline normal LVEF (>55%), during a mean follow-up of 44.2 months, only 5% of patients developed a drop in LVEF to no more than 40%, and the burden of RV pacing was not a significant multivariate predictor of LV function decrement,[13] possibly suggesting a more complex interplay of risk factors. These studies demonstrate that much remains to be learned about risk factors for the development of PICM, as discussed in the following sections.

In addition to deterioration of LV function and HF events, it has been suggested that the development of atrial fibrillation (AF) may also be a manifestation of PICM in certain patients. In a randomized trial of atrial versus dual-chamber pacing for sinus node dysfunction in 177 patients, higher burden ventricular pacing in the dual-chamber arm was associated with a significantly increased risk of AF at a mean follow-up of 2.9 years compared with atrial-only pacing (23.3 vs 7.4%, P = .03).[14] In this study, ventricular pacing was also associated with increased left atrial and ventricular volumes, suggesting a plausible mechanism for the development of AF in the setting of RV pacing. Similarly, in the aforementioned MOST study, the incidence of AF also increased in a relatively linear fashion with increased ventricular pacing burden.[8] It should be noted, however, that the incidence of AF specifically attributable to high-burden RV pacing has not been well defined, particularly given the complex interplay between cardiomyopathy and atrial arrhythmias. But given the burgeoning epidemic of AF and HF, understanding the role that PICM may play in initiating or worsening AF is an important area of investigation.

TIME COURSE OF PACING-INDUCED CARDIOMYOPATHY

As described previously, several studies have suggested that PICM begins to manifest as a drop in LVEF during the first few (approximately 1–4) years after the institution of high-burden RV pacing. However, other clinical studies suggest that the effect may be more acute. In the PACE study, a modest but significant drop in LVEF was already noted by the 12-month time point, with a decrement from 61.5% at baseline to 54.8% in the RV pacing group.[6] Although the LVEF remained in the normal range in this arm of the study, the results suggest that subtle degrees of LV dysfunction may be discernible relatively soon after the institution of RV pacing but that more clinically overt evidence of LV dysfunction (ie, LVEF <50%) may take longer to develop. In a similar vein, a significant increase in new HF diagnoses was noted within the first 6 months after presumed high-burden RV pacing in the study by Merchant and colleagues,[9] again consistent with a more acute effect and an earlier time course for the development of PICM. It is conceivable that the reported time course may vary based on whether symptoms of HF or drops in LVEF are used for the definition of PICM. Some patients may develop symptoms from ventricular dyssynchrony and elevated cardiac filling pressures before a notable drop in LVEF becomes manifest, thereby impacting the time course with which PICM is reported to occur.

POTENTIAL MECHANISMS FOR PACING-INDUCED CARDIOMYOPATHY

In general, most of the detrimental effects of RV pacing have been attributed to abnormal electrical

and mechanical activation of the ventricles, resulting in interventricular dyssynchrony and delayed activation of the basal, lateral LV (**Fig. 1**). Alterations in the normal pattern of electrical and mechanical activation result in redistribution of myocardial strain, with sites closest to the pacing site (most commonly RV apical pacing) demonstrating early systolic shortening relative to later activating segments, leading to inefficient myocardial work and impaired contractile function.[15] These effects can reduce cardiac output, increase cardiac filling pressures, and worsen functional mitral regurgitation,[16,17] all of which contribute to HF symptoms. Redistribution of myocardial work may also lead to changes in cardiac metabolism and result in regional abnormalities of myocardial perfusion, even in the absence of coronary artery disease.[15] At an ultrastructural level, myofibrillar disarray has been demonstrated within 3 months of chronic RV pacing in a dog model,[18] and degenerative fibrosis and mitochondrial abnormalities have been noted on LV biopsies from patients with congenital AV block after long-term RV pacing.[19]

In a mechanistic study of 12 patients who underwent serial assessments of LVEF via gated blood pool scans after initiation of dual-chamber pacing with short AV delay to force RV pacing, a discernible drop in LVEF was noted within 2 hours of RV pacing (60.3% vs baseline 66.5%, $P<.0002$). LV function continued to deteriorate as forced RV pacing was continued for 1 week.[20] Interestingly, although LVEF improved after the cessation of RV pacing, it remained impaired compared with baseline for over 24 hours after restoration of a normal pattern of electrical ventricular activation, suggesting that electrical dyssynchrony does not fully account for impairments in LV performance noted in the setting of RV pacing.

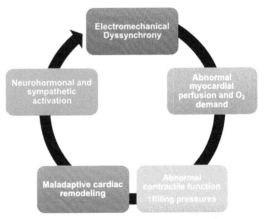

Fig. 1. Mechanisms for development of pacing-induced cardiomyopathy.

RISK FACTORS FOR PACING-INDUCED CARDIOMYOPATHY

Several single-center and limited multicenter studies have attempted to identify risk factors for developing PICM (**Box 1**). A few of the pre-RV pacing risk factors that have been identified include intrinsic QRS duration and presence of baseline LV dysfunction. Post-RV pacing risk factors include decline in global longitudinal strain, paced QRS duration, and percentage RV pacing. However, these studies have largely been limited by small sample sizes, inconsistent definitions of PICM, and variable duration of follow-up (**Table 1**).

Khurshid and colleagues[3,21] identified 1750 consecutive patients who underwent a single-chamber ventricular or dual-chamber pacemaker between 2003 and 2012. From this cohort, they identified 257 patients in whom the initial LVEF was at least 50%, a repeat echocardiogram was available at least 1 year after pacemaker implantation, and frequent (≥20%) RV pacing was present. PICM was defined as at least a 10% decrease in LVEF, resulting in an LVEF less than 50%. PICM developed in approximately 20% of patients and was observed with an RV pacing exposure as little as 20%. In multivariate analysis, male gender and a wider native QRS duration were independently associated with the development of PICM. A paced QRS duration of at least 150 milliseconds was 95% sensitive for PICM; importantly, only half of patients with PICM had HF signs or symptoms at the time of echocardiographic diagnosis.[21]

The development of PICM in patients with at least 20% RV pacing was confirmed in another study. Kiehl and colleagues[5] evaluated 823 consecutive patients who underwent a single-chamber ventricular or dual-chamber pacemaker between 2000 and 2014. All patients had complete heart block and a baseline LVEF greater than 50%. PICM was defined by need for CRT upgrade to reduction in LVEF to no more than 40%. During follow-up, approximately 12% of patients developed a PICM. In multivariate analysis, lower prepacemaker LVEF, greater RV pacing percentage, and an RV pacing percentage of at least 20% identified patients who developed PICM. Of note, upgrade to a CRT device in patients with a PICM was successful in restoring LV function in these patients.

Other investigators have sought to assess the ability of additional clinical variables to identify patients at risk for PICM. For example, Lee and colleagues[4] evaluated 234 patients who underwent a single-chamber ventricular or dual-chamber pacemaker for management of sinus node dysfunction or atrioventricular block. All patients had an LVEF greater than 40% at baseline, and none had any other documented cardiovascular disease. The electrocardiogram (ECG) was used to estimate a myocardial scar score. PICM was defined by a decrease in LVEF greater than 5% with symptoms of HF without another etiology for HF. During a mean follow-up of nearly 16 years, approximately 20% of patients developed PICM. Importantly, the mean duration from pacemaker implantation to development of HF symptoms was 13 years, highlighting the need for long-duration follow-up in these patients. In multivariate analysis, older age at implantation, a longer paced QRS duration, a higher myocardial scar score, and a higher percentage of ventricular pacing were independent predictors of pacing-induced HF. These investigators found that a paced QRS duration of at least 185 milliseconds had a 67% sensitivity and 76% specificity for detecting pacing-induced HF.

The only multicenter analysis was performed by Kim and colleagues,[22] who evaluated 130 patients (recruited at 3 centers) with complete heart block, no history of persistent or permanent atrial fibrillation, normal LVEF at baseline, and availability of pre- and postimplant echocardiograms. PICM was defined as at least a 10% decrease in LVEF, resulting in an LVEF less than 50%. During follow-up, 16% of patients developed a PICM. Risk factors for PICM included wider native QRS duration, longer baseline QTc interval, and wider paced QRS duration. In this study, a paced QRS duration of at least 140 milliseconds had a sensitivity of 95%. and a paced QRS duration of at least 167 milliseconds had a specificity of 90% for predicting the occurrence of PICM.

Box 1
Risk factors for pacing-induced cardiomyopathy

Prepacing Risk Factors

- Age
- Male gender
- Intrinsic QRS duration
- Baseline left ventricular dysfunction
- History of atrial fibrillation

Postpacing Risk Factors

- Paced QRS duration
- Decline in global longitudinal strain
- Percentage of right ventricular pacing

Table 1
Predictors of pacing induced cardiomyopathy

Study	Inclusion Criteria	Patients, n	Definition of PICM	Average Follow-up, Years	Patients with PICM, n (%)	Independent Risk Factors
Khurshid et al,[3] 2014 (single center); Khurshid et al,[21] 2016	RV single of dual chamber PPM; frequent ($\geq$20%) RV pacing; repeat echocardiogram performed $\geq$1 y post-PPM implantation	257	$\geq$10% decrease in LVEF < resulting in LVEF <50%	3.3	50 (19.5%)	Male gender (HR 2.15; 95% CI: 1.7–3.94, P = .01) Wider native QRS duration (HR 1.03 per 1 ms increase; 95% CI: 1.01–1.05, P<.001) Paced QRS $\geq$150 ms was 95% sensitive for development of PICM
Kiehl et al,[5] 2016 (single center)	RV single of dual chamber PPM; complete heart block; LVEF >50%	823	Post-PPM LVEF $\leq$40% or need for CRT upgrade	4.3	101 (12.3%)	Baseline LV dysfunction (HR 1.047 per 1% decrease; 95% CI: 1.002–1.087, P = .02) % RV pacing (HR 1.011 per 1% RV pacing; 95% CI: 1.002–1.020, P = .21) $\geq$20% RV pacing (HR: 6.76; 95% CI: 2.08–22.0, P = .002)
Lee at al,[4] 2016 (single center)	RV single of dual-chamber PPM; sinus node dysfunction or atrioventricular block; LVEF >40%	234	LVEF decrease >5% with symptoms of HF without other etiology for HF	15.6	48 (20.5%)	Old age (HR 1.62; 95% CI: 1.22–2.16, P = .001) Longer-paced QRS duration (HR 1.54; 95% CI: 1.15–2.05, P = .003) Higher myocardial scar score (HR: 1.23; 95% CI 1.03–1.49, P = .037) Higher percentage RV pacing (HR 1.31; 95% CI: 1.01–1.49, P = .010)
Kim et al,[22] 2018 (3 centers)	RV single of dual-chamber PPM; complete heart block; echocardiogram before and after PPM implantation	130	$\geq$10% decrease in LVEF < resulting in LVEF <50%	4.5	21 (16.1%)	Paced QRS duration (HR 1.05; 95% CI: 1.02–1.09, P = .001)

Abbreviations: CI, confidence interval; CRT, cardiac resynchronization therapy; HF, heart failure; HR, hazard ratio; LVEF, left ventricular ejection fraction; PICM, pacing-induced cardiomyopathy; PPM, permanent pacemaker; RV, right ventricular.

PREVENTION AND TREATMENT OF PACING-INDUCED CARDIOMYOPATHY

Several strategies have been proposed to prevent the development of PICM. One common strategy is to place the RV lead in a septal location as opposed to the traditional apical location. However, randomized clinical trials have failed to show the merits of this approach. In the PROTECT-PACE study, 240 patients with high-grade AV block, greater than 90% anticipated RV pacing, and LVEF greater than 50% were randomized to undergo pacing from the RV apex or high septal region.[23] Although it took more time and fluoroscopy to place the lead in the high septal region, there was no significant differences in HF hospitalization, mortality, the burden of atrial fibrillation, or plasma brain natriuretic peptide levels between the 2 groups.

A second strategy is to use device-based algorithms that minimize ventricular pacing. Although these algorithms are effective, it has been difficult to demonstrate a meaningful improvement in hard endpoints. A recent meta-analysis reviewed 7 randomized clinical trials that enrolled 4119 patients and compared dual-chamber pacing programmed to use minimize RV pacing algorithms with standard DDD pacing.[24] Although there was a marked reduction in the percentage of RV pacing with these algorithms, during a mean follow-up of 2.5 years there were no differences in likelihood of developing persistent atrial fibrillation, all-cause hospitalization, or all-cause mortality between the 2 groups. Furthermore, there remains a concern about the impact of excessively prolonged PR intervals when using these types of pacing algorithms. In a study of patients receiving a dual-chamber ICD, a ventricular pacing algorithm that minimized the percentage of ventricular pacing was associated with more HF and worse outcomes in patients with a PR interval of at least 230 milliseconds. It has been suggested the adverse hemodynamic effects of long PR intervals, through prolonged intrinsic AV conduction, including shortening and impairment of LV filling and increased left atrial pressure; these adverse effects may be particularly clinically meaningful in patients with decreased LV function.[25]

A third strategy is to implant a cardiac resynchronization therapy device from the onset. This strategy has been tested in 2 randomized clinical trials. The BIOPACE study (Biventricular Pacing for Atrioventricular Block to Prevent Cardiac Desynchronization) enrolled only few patients with either a PR interval greater than 230 milliseconds or complete heart block.[26] The trial failed to demonstrate that biventricular pacing was better than standard RV pacing with respect to its primary objective (mortality and HF hospitalization) during a mean follow-up of 67 months. On the other hand, the BLOCK-HF study (Biventricular vs Right Ventricular Pacing in Heart Failure

Table 2
Ongoing randomized clinical trials of His-bundle pacing

Study	Centers	Anticipated Enrollment	Randomization	Primary Outcome
His bundle pacing vs CS pacing for CRT (His-SYNC) (NCT02700425)	University of Chicago Geisinger Indiana Northwestern University of California Los Angeles	n = 40 (HF, EF ≤35%, QRS >120 ms, and class I or IIa CRT indication)	HBP vs CRT	• Change in EF • Change in QRS duration • Time to 1st CV hospitalization or death
Comparison of His bundle and BiV pacing in HF with AF (NCT02805465)	First Affiliated Hospital Wenzhou Medical University	n = 50 (persistent AF/ flutter, HF, EF <40%)	AVJ + CRT (HB lead in A port) HBP vs CRT, crossover study	• Change of EF from baseline
The His optimized pacing evaluated for HF trial (HOPE-HF) (NCT02671903)	Imperial College London	n = 160 (HF, EF <35%, PR ≥200 ms, QRS ≤140 ms or RBBB)	CRT (HB lead in all patients) No pacing vs HBP	• Change in exercise capacity

Abbreviations: A, atrial; AF, atrial fibrillation; AVJ, atrioventricular junction; BiV, biventricular; CRT, cardiac resynchronization therapy; CS, coronary sinus; CV, cardiovascular; EF, ejection fraction; HBP, his-bundle pacing; HF, heart failure; RBBB, right bundle branch block.

Patients with Atrioventricular Block) did meet its primary end point and showed that biventricular pacing reduces the risk of all-cause mortality, HF-related urgent care visits, or an increase of at least 15% in LV end-systolic volume index for patients with AV block and systolic dysfunction.[27] However, the end point was exclusively driven by changes in LV end systolic volume and not the clinical end points. There are concerns about routinely implanting biventricular pacemakers in these patients, unless there is existing LV dysfunction, because of the additional hardware, time needed to implant, associated complications, and implications for battery longevity.

The fourth strategy appears to be the most promising, namely, to implant these patients with a His-bundle pacemaker system. The advantage of this approach is that its remains a dual-chamber pacemaker, whereby the ventricular lead is placed directly onto the His bundle (using the lead itself to map and locate the His-bundle). By selectively engaging the His-bundle system, pacing fails to induce the dyssynchrony that is inherent to RV septal or apical pacing. Recently, His-bundle pacing has been shown to be feasible in a high percentage of patients exposed to a high burden of RV pacing and resulting LV dysfunction and HF.[28] During follow-up, pacing resulted in LV reverse remodeling and improved clinical outcomes in PICM patients. Several small randomized clinical trials are currently underway to formally assess the safety and efficacy of His-bundle pacing in a variety of clinical settings (**Table 2**). In particular, data are needed to

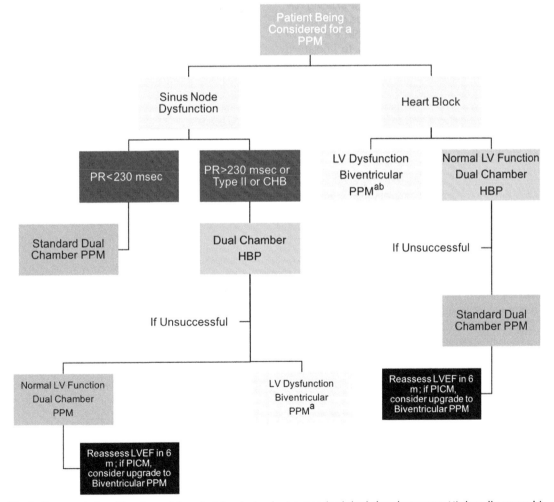

Fig. 2. Proposed algorithm for guiding decision to implant a standard dual chamber versus His-bundle versus biventricular pacemaker in a patient with sinus node dysfunction or heart block. CHB, complete heart block; HBP, his-bundle pacemaker; ICD, implantable cardioverter-defibrillator; LV, left ventricular; LVEF, LV ejection fraction; PICM, pacing-induced cardiomyopathy; PPM, permanent pacemaker. [a] Assess for need for ICD implantation. [b] Can consider HBP if unsuccessful at attempt to implant a biventricular PPM.

determine the acute procedural success rates in patients with excessively prolonged PR intervals and advanced heart block, long-term stability of the lead anatomically and with respect to electrical performance, and the ability to mitigate development of PICM.

SUMMARY

In summary, after decades of RV pacing, it is clear that some patients will develop a PICM. However, many individuals tolerate high-burden RV burden well for many years, and physicians are still challenged by their inability to reliably identify patients most likely to develop a PICM. For many reasons, routine implantation of a biventricular pacemaker in patients likely to be exposed to a high burden of RV pacing has not emerged as a standard of care, unless patients have pre-existing LV dysfunction. His-bundle pacing holds great promise, because it may be able to avoid the risk of PICM while allowing the physician to implant a dual-chamber pacing system. Thus, until more data become available, the authors propose an approach that is summarized in **Fig. 2**. The authors feel that this may offer clinicians the best practical opportunity to prevent and treat PICM.

REFERENCES

1. Mond HG, Proclemer A. The 11th world survey of cardiac pacing and implantable cardioverter-defibrillators: calendar year 2009–a World Society of Arrhythmia's project. Pacing Clin Electrophysiol 2011;34:1013–27.

2. Chen L, Hodge D, Jahangir A, et al. Preserved left ventricular ejection fraction following atrioventricular junction ablation and pacing for atrial fibrillation. J Cardiovasc Electrophysiol 2008;19:19–27.

3. Khurshid S, Epstein AE, Verdino RJ, et al. Incidence and predictors of right ventricular pacing-induced cardiomyopathy. Heart Rhythm 2014;11:1619–25.

4. Lee SA, Cha MJ, Cho Y, et al. Paced QRS duration and myocardial scar amount: predictors of long-term outcome of right ventricular apical pacing. Heart Vessels 2016;31:1131–9.

5. Kiehl EL, Makki T, Kumar R, et al. Incidence and predictors of right ventricular pacing-induced cardiomyopathy in patients with complete atrioventricular block and preserved left ventricular systolic function. Heart Rhythm 2016;13:2272–8.

6. Yu CM, Chan JY, Zhang Q, et al. Biventricular pacing in patients with bradycardia and normal ejection fraction. N Engl J Med 2009;361:2123–34.

7. Yu CM, Fang F, Luo XX, et al. Long-term follow-up results of the pacing to avoid cardiac enlargement (PACE) trial. Eur J Heart Fail 2014;16:1016–25.

8. Sweeney MO, Hellkamp AS, Ellenbogen KA, et al. Adverse effect of ventricular pacing on heart failure and atrial fibrillation among patients with normal baseline QRS duration in a clinical trial of pacemaker therapy for sinus node dysfunction. Circulation 2003;107:2932–7.

9. Merchant FM, Hoskins MH, Musat DL, et al. Incidence and time course for developing heart failure with high-burden right ventricular pacing. Circ Cardiovasc Qual Outcomes 2017;10 [pii:e003564].

10. Curtis AB, Worley SJ, Chung ES, et al. Improvement in clinical outcomes with biventricular versus right ventricular pacing: the BLOCK HF study. J Am Coll Cardiol 2016;67:2148–57.

11. Sharma AD, Rizo-Patron C, Hallstrom AP, et al. Percent right ventricular pacing predicts outcomes in the DAVID trial. Heart Rhythm 2005;2:830–4.

12. Steinberg JS, Fischer A, Wang P, et al. The clinical implications of cumulative right ventricular pacing in the multicenter automatic defibrillator trial II. J Cardiovasc Electrophysiol 2005;16:359–65.

13. Ebert M, Jander N, Minners J, et al. Long-term impact of right ventricular pacing on left ventricular systolic function in pacemaker recipients with preserved ejection fraction: results from a large single-center registry. J Am Heart Assoc 2016;5 [pii:e003485].

14. Nielsen JC, Kristensen L, Andersen HR, et al. A randomized comparison of atrial and dual-chamber pacing in 177 consecutive patients with sick sinus syndrome: echocardiographic and clinical outcome. J Am Coll Cardiol 2003;42:614–23.

15. Tops LF, Schalij MJ, Bax JJ. The effects of right ventricular apical pacing on ventricular function and dyssynchrony implications for therapy. J Am Coll Cardiol 2009;54:764–76.

16. Leclercq C, Gras D, Le Helloco A, et al. Hemodynamic importance of preserving the normal sequence of ventricular activation in permanent cardiac pacing. Am Heart J 1995;129:1133–41.

17. Guglin M, Barold SS. The role of biventricular pacing in the prevention and therapy of pacemaker-induced cardiomyopathy. Ann Noninvasive Electrocardiol 2015;20:224–39.

18. Adomian GE, Beazell J. Myofibrillar disarray produced in normal hearts by chronic electrical pacing. Am Heart J 1986;112:79–83.

19. Karpawich PP, Rabah R, Haas JE. Altered cardiac histology following apical right ventricular pacing in patients with congenital atrioventricular block. Pacing Clin Electrophysiol 1999;22:1372–7.

20. Nahlawi M, Waligora M, Spies SM, et al. Left ventricular function during and after right ventricular pacing. J Am Coll Cardiol 2004;44:1883–8.

21. Khurshid S, Liang JJ, Owens A, et al. Longer paced QRS duration is associated with increased prevalence of right ventricular pacing-induced

cardiomyopathy. J Cardiovasc Electrophysiol 2016; 27:1174–9.

22. Kim JH, Kang KW, Chin JY, et al. Major determinant of the occurrence of pacing-induced cardiomyopathy in complete atrioventricular block: a multicentre, retrospective analysis over a 15-year period in South Korea. BMJ Open 2018;8:e019048.

23. Kaye GC, Linker NJ, Marwick TH, et al. Effect of right ventricular pacing lead site on left ventricular function in patients with high grade atrioventricular block: results of the Protect-Pace study. Eur Heart J 2015;36:856–62.

24. Shurrab M, Healey JS, Haj-Yahia S, et al. Reduction in unncessary ventricular pacing fails to affect hard clinical outcomes in patients with preserved left ventricular function: a meta-analysis. Europace 2017; 19:282–8.

25. Aurricchio A, Ellenbogen KA. Reducing ventricular pacing frequency in patients with atrioventricular block. Is it time to change the current pacing paradigm? Circ Arrhythm Electrophysiol 2016;9: e004404.

26. Funck RC, Mueller HH, Lunati M, et al, for the Bio-Pace study group. Characteristics of a large sample of candidates for permanent ventricular pacing included in the Biventricular Pacing for Atrioventricular Block to Prevent Cardiac Desynchronization Study (BioPace). Europace 2014;16:354–62.

27. Curtis AB, Worley SJ, Adamson PB, et al, for the Biventricular versus Right Ventricular Pacing in Heart Failure Patients with Atrioventricular Block (BLOCK HF) Trial Investigators. Biventricular pacing for atrioventricular block and systolic dysfunction. N Engl J Med 2013;368:1585–93.

28. Shan P, Su L, Zhou X, et al. Beneficial effects of upgrading to His bundle pacing in chronically paced patients with left ventricular ejection fraction < 50%. Heart Rhythm 2018;15:405–12.

Tricuspid Valve Dysfunction Caused by Right Ventricular Leads

Elisa Ebrille, MD, James D. Chang, MD,
Peter J. Zimetbaum, MD*

KEYWORDS

- Tricuspid regurgitation • Tricuspid valve • Right ventricular leads • Lead-related dysfunction

KEY POINTS

- Tricuspid regurgitation (TR) is increasingly recognized as a clinically significant valvular condition.
- The role of multiple pacemaker and implantable cardiac defibrillator leads in distortion of the valve structure and the risk of trauma to the valve and subvalvular apparatus with lead extraction contribute to the development of TR.
- There is a clinical imperative to better understand the optimal way to diagnose lead-related TR, risk factors for the development of TR, and optimal strategies to mitigate this problem.

INTRODUCTION

The vast majority of cardiovascular implantable electronic devices (CIEDs) require a ventricular lead to be placed across the tricuspid valve (TV). TV dysfunction caused by the presence of a right ventricular (RV) lead crossing the valve has not been a well-recognized entity until recently. The contribution of device leads to tricuspid regurgitation (TR) has gained increasing recognition with the development of advanced imaging techniques, such as 3-dimensional (3D) echocardiography, which more accurately assess the interaction of the ventricular lead with the TV apparatus.

TRICUSPID VALVE DYSFUNCTION CAUSED BY RIGHT VENTRICULAR LEADS

Tricuspid Valve

Although historically being the "neglected" valve, the tricuspid apparatus has a complex structure whose proper function is strictly dependent on the interaction among several different components.

The TV is the most anteriorly located of the heart valves, with a nearly vertical orientation within the heart. Its orifice has an oval shape and is larger than that of the mitral valve. It is composed of 3 leaflets unequal in size (anterior, posterior, and septal), chordae tendineae, and 2 papillary muscles (anterior and posterior). The leaflets and chordae tendineae are thinner than those of the mitral valve and, unlike the mitral apparatus, some of the TV chordae tendineae attach directly to the interventricular septum, ventricular free wall, or moderator band in the absence of an intervening papillary muscle. Most frequently, TR is caused by RV pressure/volume overload (and therefore described as functional, or secondary), leading to annular dilation, leaflet tethering, and loss of coaptation. Intuitively, the presence of a CIED lead, interfering with valve closure and possibly damaging the valvular and subvalvular apparatus, can significantly worsen the TR and result in consequent morbidity. In many cases, the presence of a lead across the TV plays a permissive role in exacerbating functional TR that might otherwise have

Department of Medicine, Cardiovascular Division, Beth Israel Deaconess Medical Center, Harvard Medical School, 185 Pilgrim Road, Baker 4, Boston, MA, 02215, USA
* Corresponding author. Department of Medicine, Cardiovascular Division, Beth Israel Deaconess Medical Center, Harvard Medical School, 185 Pilgrim Road, Baker 4, Boston, MA 02215.
E-mail address: pzimetba@bidmc.harvard.edu

Card Electrophysiol Clin 10 (2018) 447–452
https://doi.org/10.1016/j.ccep.2018.05.006

been less severe. Major adverse consequences stemming independently from lead-induced TV dysfunction with respect to both mortality and morbidity have been abundantly documented.[1–5]

Mechanisms of Lead-Related Dysfunction

Lead-related TV dysfunction can occur by several direct and indirect mechanisms. These include mechanical valve obstruction caused by the presence of the lead in between the leaflets (impingement), fibrotic attachment between lead and leaflet(s) causing closure impairment, lead entanglement with TV support structures, leaflet perforation, laceration, and even avulsion.[6–11] Procedural and technical factors can affect the type and probability of valve damage during lead advancement and positioning. Among the 3 common modalities to place an RV lead,[12] the "prolapsing technique" may theoretically reduce the risk of perforation and laceration compared with the "direct crossing technique" and the "drop-down technique," because of less direct head-on trauma on the TV and subvalvular apparatus. Moreover, because the TV leaflets are not seen on fluoroscopy, determining the lead position in relation to the TV leaflets at the time of implant is challenging. The type of lead-tip fixation mechanism can also affect the probability of TV damage, the passive fixation leads (tined leads) associated with higher potential risk of perforation, or laceration of the TV and subvalvular apparatus compared with active fixation leads (screw-in leads), either at implant or during a lead extraction procedure.[13–15]

The mere presence of a foreign body traversing the TV, interfering with normal tricuspid leaflet coaptation and valve closure by direct interaction with the valve leaflets (impingement) or by entanglement with the chordae tendineae can result in TR. Although Seo and colleagues[16] demonstrated that most TR in patients with transvalvular leads occurred when the lead was located between the posterior and the septal tricuspid leaflet, Krupa and colleagues[17] did not show an association between the location of the lead at the level of the tricuspid orifice and TR severity. A study from Al-Bawardy and colleagues[18] demonstrated that leads placed in an apical position are associated with an increased risk of tethering to the posterior leaflet compared with septally placed leads.

Theoretically, direct lead interference with valve closure should proportionally increase with the number of implanted leads.[19] Postaci and colleagues[20] showed that the incidence of TR was more frequent and of higher degree in patients with 2 leads compared with patients with a single lead device. A series from de Cock and colleagues[21] confirmed that having multiple pacemaker (PM) leads across the TV correlates with echocardiographic finding of significant TR. A recent large single-center longitudinal cohort analysis[1] showed that the prevalence of significant TR is higher in patients with a PM compared with patients without a PM after adjustment for left ventricular systolic and diastolic function and pulmonary artery hypertension and is associated with an increased mortality risk.

Even more debatable is the relationship between lead composition and TV damage. Lin and colleagues[6] demonstrated a trend toward the increased development of TR in patients with silicone-coated leads compared with polyurethane leads. However, due to small sample size, a conclusive statement regarding a definite relationship between lead composition and TR could not be drawn.

In addition to small sample size, most published studies include mixed samples of patients with a device, making no distinction between PM and implantable cardiac defibrillator (ICD) leads. Prevalence of significant TR, defined as $\geq$2, and incidence of worsening TR by 1 or more grades following device implantation varies from 10% to 39%, with most (but not all) studies attributing a higher incidence of worsening TR to ICD leads.[7,8,16–18,20–27] A study from Kim and colleagues,[7] including 248 patients with either ICD or PM, showed that TR was more common in patients with ICD leads compared with PM leads (32.4% vs 20.7%, $P = .048$). The greater thickness and stiffness of the more rigid ICD lead have been implicated as the causative mechanism. Discordant data may derive from the fact that the greater thickness of ICD leads compared with PM leads is also responsible for a greater echocardiographic acoustic artifact, resulting in Doppler color flow signal attenuation and TR underestimation. On the other hand, patients with ICDs usually have at least moderate to severe left ventricular dysfunction and are thereby predisposed to a greater degree of functional TR compared with patients with PM leads and without left ventricular dysfunction.

Another mechanism of lead-related TR dysfunction, intuitively more frequent in ICD leads, is the foreign body fibrotic and inflammatory response that can occur as early as 12 hours postprocedure.[9] Chronic repetitive contact between device leads and leaflet or chordal structures results in neoendocardium formation and development of a fibrin sheath that can extend along the entire endovascular course of the lead. This results in encapsulation, ensheathment, or entrapment of the lead with subsequent loss of leaflet mobility or coaptation.[28–37] Thrombosis along the lead or at the site of electrode implantation also may occur 4 to 5 days after lead positioning.[38] Organization of thrombi around the leads, however, is not always associated with TR development or worsening.

Along with the worldwide increase in number of PM and ICD implantations has come a rise in the rates of device and lead failure and complications, notably infection, which is increasing faster than the rate of implantations.[39] This is due in part to the growing number of implantations in elderly patients with multiple comorbidities and therefore a higher risk of sepsis or endocarditis. Device infection, or even the mere presence of bacteremia in a patient with a device, is associated with significant mortality (particularly if the TV itself is involved), morbidity, and health care expenditure, with necessity for expeditious device and lead extraction.[40] It has been estimated that 24,000 transvenous lead extractions (TLEs) occur annually worldwide,[41] with device infection being the indication in two-thirds of the cases.[42] Because of the tendency of TV leaflet or subvalvular apparatus to adhere to and/or encapsulate PM and ICD leads over time, TLE can result in major TV apparatus damage.

Current lead extraction techniques include mechanical and laser-assisted dissection rather than manual traction of the lead, with a reported decreased incidence of worsening TR (0% to 5.6%) and higher procedural success than in the past (94% to 100%).[43–45] Franceschi and colleagues[46] prospectively evaluated 208 patients who underwent removal of 237 ventricular leads. They used a stepwise approach, starting with gentle traction applied on the lead from the pocket, followed by laser sheath or lasso tools. They observed a 9.1% rate of traumatic TR and, after multivariate analysis, found female sex and the use of additional tools, such as lasso or laser sheath, to be independent predictors of traumatic TR. At a median follow-up of 17.9 months, patients who developed TR had high incidence of right-sided heart failure symptoms without a significant increase in overall mortality. However, as suggested by the study of Delling and colleagues,[1] there can be little doubt that longer follow-up would have disclosed a significant incremental mortality from lead-related TR. Female gender was again a predictor of significant TR in a series of 311 patients and 552 leads removed with manual traction or laser.[47] The investigators postulated that the reason for their finding was the tendency for increased fibrosis development in the female population. Moreover, the use of laser did not predict the development of significant TR. The initial idea that laser sheath–assisted extractions were characterized by a higher risk of TV damage[45,46,48]

more likely reflects a higher degree of lead entrapment requiring a more aggressive approach with laser, rather than a shortcoming of the laser technique. A retrospective analysis from a prospectively collected database of 86 patients, in whom laser sheaths were not used and leads were extracted with manual traction or with mechanical and powered sheaths, showed an increase of at least 1 grade in TR in 15.1% of the patients.[49] Young age at extraction (increased inflammatory response and fibrosis in younger compared with older individuals) and use of mechanical sheaths were the only 2 identified factors that predicted TR worsening, regardless the type of the lead, the number of leads, and time since implantation.

Diagnosis of Lead-Related Tricuspid Valve Damage

As in any other challenging medical scenario, to diagnose lead-related TR, one has to first acknowledge its possibility and to maintain a high index of clinical suspicion based on the patient's history and physical examination. The contribution of device leads to TV damage/dysfunction has started to gain recognition only in the more recent years. This is because historically 2D echocardiography has been the mainstay of real-time cardiac imaging.

The TV is not easily imaged by 2D echocardiography, because an en face view of the valve simultaneously displaying all 3 leaflets usually is not possible.[50,51] Multiple views are required to assess the TV and no more than 2 leaflets are displayed in any one view. Moreover, following the entire lead course, from the point at which it crosses the TV annulus down to its juxtaposition with the subvalvular apparatus, is not feasible. In a study by Seo and colleagues,[16] in only 15 of 87 patients with a device was 2D echocardiography able to correctly identify the course of a lead through the valve when compared with 3D echocardiography (see later in this article). A major pitfall of 2D echocardiography remains the underestimation of TR severity due to the presence of acoustic shadowing and scattering that lead to Doppler signal attenuation. Moreover, the TR jet itself may be obscured by the physical presence of the lead. In most cases, especially when the damage on the valve is caused by valve tethering or asymmetrical leaflet mobility, the TR jet tends to be eccentric, resulting in the Coanda effect (tendency of a fluid to stay attached to a convex surface, the wall of the right atrium in this case) and loss of Doppler color flow signal. In a study from Lin and colleagues[6] on patients who eventually were found to have severe lead-induced TR intraoperatively, only 26 (63%) of 41 cases received a correct diagnosis with the preoperative 2D transthoracic echocardiography. Last, the systolic pressure gradient between the RV and the right atrium may be very small in the setting of severe TR, leading to a resultant low TR velocity and underestimation of the jet area. Indirect measurements of TR severity that are not affected by lead-induced acoustic artifacts, such as the examination of the hepatic vein flow (presence of holosystolic hepatic vein flow reversal is diagnostic of severe TR, except in the case of a massively dilated right atrium), can be helpful and should be routinely performed in all patients with CIEDs. Two-dimensional transesophageal echocardiography offers better images compared with 2D transthoracic echocardiography, but still cannot display all 3 TV leaflets in a single view.

Three-dimensional echocardiography, which provides full-volume views of cardiac structures, should be the imaging modality of choice in patients with CIEDs. Three-dimensional echocardiography can indeed visualize the TV en face, allowing simultaneous visualization of the 3 leaflets, their movements, valve coaptation, potential lead impingement, and lead course (**Fig. 1**). Seo and colleagues[16] reported 94.2% sensitivity of 3D echocardiography in identifying the course of the lead and its location at the TV annulus compared with 17.2% sensitivity when 2D echocardiography was used. Other second-level imaging modalities, such as chest computed tomography and cardiac MRI, can be sometimes contraindicated and are still characterized by inadequate images due to artifacts from the endocardial lead.

Treatment of Lead-Related Tricuspid Valve Damage

Once the severity of TR and RV enlargement and dysfunction are confirmed and the role of the lead interfering with TV mobility and or coaptation have been documented, TLE ± TV repair or replacement should be considered. Sometimes lead extraction alone without valve repair or replacement can be enough to correct TR, especially if the lead is relatively new and the damage to the valvular and subvalvular apparatus is negligible. However, in a considerable number of cases, corrective surgical treatment is necessary. Suture annuloplasty, ring annuloplasty, and valve replacement are the 3 modalities of choice. Suture annuloplasty implies preservation of the lead and its relocation in a cleft of the valve created by suture. Ring annuloplasty can be performed with a C-ring rather than an O-ring to allow preservation of the lead without its entrapment outside the ring itself. Valve replacement without removing the lead implies that the lead will be entrapped outside the replacement valve. Aside from the potential lead damage, this technique precludes the possibility of future lead extraction without open heart surgery. Therefore, when possible, percutaneous lead extraction should be performed first, leaving TV repair or replacement as a second step in case of absence of TV function recovery.[52]

SUMMARY

TR is increasingly recognized as a clinically significant valvular condition. The role of PM and ICD leads in distortion of the valve structure and the

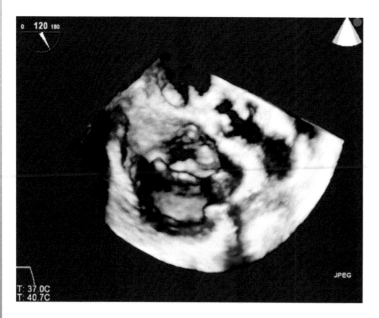

Fig. 1. Three-dimensional transesophageal echocardiogram (TEE) still-frame (at end-systole) displaying ICD lead encapsulated by posterior leaflet of TV. The septal (top and right) and anterior (bottom) leaflets exhibited minimally reduced mobility but the posterior leaflet is immobilized due to its interaction (consisting of encapsulation, fibrosis, and retraction) with the lead, resulting in a gaping regurgitant orifice.

risk of trauma to the valve and subvalvular apparatus with lead extraction contribute to the development of TR. There is a clinical imperative to better understand the optimal way to diagnose lead-related TR, risk factors for the development of TR, and optimal strategies to mitigate this problem.

REFERENCES

1. Delling FN, Hassan ZK, Piatkowski G, et al. Tricuspid regurgitation and mortality in patients with transvenous permanent pacemaker leads. Am J Cardiol 2016;117(6):988–92.

2. Höke U, Auger D, Thijssen J, et al. Significant lead-induced tricuspid regurgitation is associated with poor prognosis at long-term follow-up. Heart 2014; 100(12):960–8.

3. Al-Bawardy R, Krishnaswamy A, Rajeswaran J, et al. Tricuspid regurgitation and implantable devices. Pacing Clin Electrophysiol 2015;38(2):259–66.

4. Dilaveris P, Pantazis A, Giannopoulos G, et al. Upgrade to biventricular pacing in patients with pacing-induced heart failure: can resynchronization do the trick? Europace 2006;8(5):352–7.

5. Ebrille E, DeSimone CV, Vaidya VR, et al. Ventricular pacing—electromechanical consequences and valvular function. Indian Pacing Electrophysiol J 2016;16(1):19–30.

6. Lin G, Nishimura RA, Connolly HM, et al. Severe symptomatic tricuspid valve regurgitation due to permanent pacemaker or implantable cardioverter-defibrillator leads. J Am Coll Cardiol 2005;45(10):1672–5.

7. Kim JB, Spevack DM, Tunick PA, et al. The effect of transvenous pacemaker and implantable cardioverter defibrillator lead placement on tricuspid valve function: an observational study. J Am Soc Echocardiogr 2008;21(3):284–7.

8. Klutstein M, Balkin J, Butnaru A, et al. Tricuspid incompetence following permanent pacemaker implantation. Pacing Clin Electrophysiol 2009;32(Suppl 1):S135–7.

9. Robboy SJ, Harthorne JW, Leinbach RC, et al. Autopsy findings with permanent pervenous pacemakers. Circulation 1969;39(4):495–501.

10. Rainer PP, Schmidt A, Anelli-Monti M, et al. A swinging pacemaker lead promoting endocarditis and severe tricuspid regurgitation. J Am Coll Cardiol 2012;59(23):e45.

11. Iezzi F, Cini R, Sordini P. Tricuspid-valve repair for pacemaker leads endocarditis. BMJ Case Rep 2010;2010 [pii:bcr0120102673].

12. Rajappan K. Permanent pacemaker implantation technique: part II. Heart 2009;95(4):334–42.

13. Frandsen F, Oxhøj H, Nielsen B. Entrapment of a tined pacemaker electrode in the tricuspid valve. A case report. Pacing Clin Electrophysiol 1990;13(9): 1082–3.

14. Res JC, De Cock CC, Van Rossum AC, et al. Entrapment of tined leads. Pacing Clin Electrophysiol 1989; 12(10):1583–5.

15. Fürstenberg S, Bluhm G, Olin C. Entrapment of an atrial tined pacemaker electrode in the tricuspid valve–a case report. Pacing Clin Electrophysiol 1984;7(4):760–2.

16. Seo Y, Ishizu T, Nakajima H, et al. Clinical utility of 3-dimensional echocardiography in the evaluation of tricuspid regurgitation caused by pacemaker leads. Circ J 2008;72(9):1465–70.

17. Krupa W, Kozłowski D, Derejko P, et al. Permanent cardiac pacing and its influence on tricuspid valve function. Folia Morphol (Warsz) 2001;60(4):249–57.

18. Al-Bawardy R, Krishnaswamy A, Bhargava M, et al. Tricuspid regurgitation in patients with pacemakers and implantable cardiac defibrillators: a comprehensive review. Clin Cardiol 2013;36(5):249–54.

19. Shandling AH, Lehmann KG, Atwood JE, et al. Prevalence of catheter-induced valvular regurgitation as determined by Doppler echocardiography. Am J Cardiol 1989;63(18):1369–74.

20. Postaci N, Ekşi K, Bayata S, et al. Effect of the number of ventricular leads on right ventricular hemodynamics in patients with permanent pacemaker. Effect of the number of ventricular leads on right ventricular hemodynamics in patients with permanent pacemaker. Angiology 1995;46(5):421–4.

21. de Cock CC, Vinkers M, Van Campe LC, et al. Long-term outcome of patients with multiple (> or = 3) noninfected transvenous leads: a clinical and echocardiographic study. Pacing Clin Electrophysiol 2000;23(4 Pt 1):423–6.

22. Paniagua D, Aldrich HR, Lieberman EH, et al. Increased prevalence of significant tricuspid regurgitation in patients with transvenous pacemakers leads. Am J Cardiol 1998;82(9):1130–2. A9.

23. Barclay JL, Cross SJ, Leslie SJ. Entanglement of passive fix ventricular lead in tricuspid valve. Pacing Clin Electrophysiol 2008;31(1):138.

24. Lee RC, Friedman SE, Kono AT, et al. Tricuspid regurgitation following implantation of endocardial leads: incidence and predictors. Pacing Clin Electrophysiol 2015;38(11):1267–74.

25. Webster G, Margossian R, Alexander ME, et al. Impact of transvenous ventricular pacing leads on tricuspid regurgitation in pediatric and congenital heart disease patients. J Interv Card Electrophysiol 2008;21(1):65–8.

26. Dokainish H, Elbarasi E, Masiero S, et al. Prospective study of tricuspid valve regurgitation associated with permanent leads in patients undergoing cardiac rhythm device implantation: background, rationale, and design. Glob Cardiol Sci Pract 2015; 2015(3):41.

27. Baquero GA, Yadav P, Skibba JB, et al. Clinical significance of increased tricuspid valve incompetence

following implantation of ventricular leads. J Interv Card Electrophysiol 2013;38(3):197–202.

28. Epstein AE, Kay GN, Plumb VJ, et al. Gross and microscopic pathological changes associated with nonthoracotomy implantable defibrillator leads. Circulation 1998;98(15):1517–24.

29. Friedberg HD, D'Cunha GF. Adhesions of pacing catheter to tricuspid valve: adhesive endocarditis. Thorax 1969;24(4):498–9.

30. Stokes K, Anderson J, McVenes R, et al. The encapsulation of polyurethane-insulated transvenous cardiac pacemaker leads. Cardiovasc Pathol 1995; 4(3):163–71.

31. Candinas R, Duru F, Schneider J, et al. Postmortem analysis of encapsulation around long-term ventricular endocardial pacing leads. Mayo Clin Proc 1999; 74(2):120–5.

32. Myers MR, Parsonnet V, Bernstein AD. Extraction of implanted transvenous pacing leads: a review of a persistent clinical problem. Am Heart J 1991;121(3 Pt 1):881–8.

33. Iskandar SB, Ann Jackson S, Fahrig S, et al. Tricuspid valve malfunction and ventricular pacemaker lead: case report and review of the literature. Echocardiography 2006;23(8):692–7.

34. Taira K, Suzuki A, Fujino A, et al. Tricuspid valve stenosis related to subvalvular adhesion of pacemaker lead: a case report. J Cardiol 2006;47(6):301–6.

35. Heaven DJ, Henein MY, Sutton R. Pacemaker lead related tricuspid stenosis: a report of two cases. Heart 2000;83(3):351–2.

36. Nisanci Y, Yilmaz E, Oncul A, et al. Predominant tricuspid stenosis secondary to bacterial endocarditis in a patient with permanent pacemaker and balloon dilatation of the stenosis. Pacing Clin Electrophysiol 1999;22(2):393–6.

37. Old WD, Paulsen W, Lewis SA, et al. Pacemaker lead-induced tricuspid stenosis: diagnosis by Doppler echocardiography. Am Heart J 1989;117(5):1165–7.

38. Huang TY, Baba N. Cardiac pathology of transvenous pacemakers. Am Heart J 1972;83(4):469–74.

39. Voigt A, Shalaby A, Saba S. Continued rise in rates of cardiovascular implantable electronic device infections in the United States: temporal trends and causative insights. Pacing Clin Electrophysiol 2010;33(4):414–9.

40. Athan E, Chu VH, Tattevin P, et al, ICE-PCS Investigators. Clinical characteristics and outcome of infective endocarditis involving implantable cardiac devices. JAMA 2012;307(16):1727–35.

41. Maytin M, Daily TP, Carillo RG. Virtual reality lead extraction as a method for training new physicians: a pilot study. Pacing Clin Electrophysiol 2015; 38(3):319–25.

42. Di Monaco A, Pelargonio G, Narducci ML, et al. Safety of transvenous lead extraction according to centre volume: a systematic review and meta-analysis. Europace 2014;16(10):1496–507.

43. Byrd CL, Wilkoff BL, Love CJ, et al. Intravascular extraction of problematic or infected permanent pacemaker leads: 1994-1996. U.S. extraction database, MED Institute. Pacing Clin Electrophysiol 1999;22(9):1348–57.

44. Rodriguez Y, Mesa J, Arguelles E, et al. Tricuspid insufficiency after laser lead extraction. Pacing Clin Electrophysiol 2013;36(8):939–44.

45. Coffey JO, Sager SJ, Gangireddy S, et al. The impact of transvenous lead extraction on tricuspid valve function. Pacing Clin Electrophysiol 2014; 37(1):19–24.

46. Franceschi F, Thuny F, Giorgi R, et al. Incidence, risk factors, and outcome of traumatic tricuspid regurgitation after percutaneous ventricular lead removal. J Am Coll Cardiol 2009;53(23):2168–74.

47. Glover BM, Watkins S, Mariani JA, et al. Prevalence of tricuspid regurgitation and pericardial effusions following pacemaker and defibrillator lead extraction. Int J Cardiol 2010;145(3):593–4.

48. Roeffel S, Bracke F, Meijer A, et al. Transesophageal echocardiographic evaluation of tricuspid valve regurgitation during pacemaker and implantable cardioverter defibrillator lead extraction. Pacing Clin Electrophysiol 2002;25(11):1583–6.

49. Givon A, Vedernikova N, Luria D, et al. Tricuspid regurgitation following lead extraction: risk factors and clinical course. Isr Med Assoc J 2016;18(1): 18–22.

50. Badano LP, Agricola E, Perez de Isla L, et al. Evaluation of the tricuspid valve morphology and function by transthoracic real-time three-dimensional echocardiography. Eur J Echocardiogr 2009;10(4):477–84.

51. Muraru D, Badano LP, Sarais C, et al. Evaluation of tricuspid valve morphology and function by transthoracic three-dimensional echocardiography. Curr Cardiol Rep 2011;13(3):242–9.

52. Chang JD, Manning WJ, Ebrille E, et al. Tricuspid valve dysfunction following pacemaker or cardioverter-defibrillator implantation. J Am Coll Cardiol 2017;69(18):2331–41.

His Bundle Pacing
Concept to Reality

Pramod Deshmukh, MD

KEYWORDS

• His bundle pacing • Right ventricular pacing • Pacing-induced cardiomyopathy

KEY POINTS

- The properties of the His bundle and adjacent tissues allows for a precise electrophysiologic definition of selective His bundle pacing in patients with nondiseased His Purkinje conduction systems.
- Several key technologies have made the His bundle a feasible, safe, and effective site for permanent pacing.
- His bundle pacing has potential applications in a wide variety of clinical scenarios.

INITIAL EXPERIENCE: ABLATE AND PACE IN ATRIAL FIBRILLATION AND HEART FAILURE

The author's first experience with permanent His bundle pacing (HBP), which was reported at the Heart Rhythm Society in 1995, occurred when presented with a patient who was referred for tachycardia-induced cardiomyopathy and atrial fibrillation (AF) refractory to pharmacologic therapy.[1] The patient was critically ill with ejection fraction of 10%, functional class IV, and was dependent on dopamine therapy. At this time, the concept of tachycardia-induced cardiomyopathy and its reversal by either surgical or radiofrequency ablation was well known.[2,3] In addition, rate control of refractory AF via atrioventricular (AV) nodal ablation and pacemaker placement had been associated with improved functional status.[4]

However, evidence of the deleterious effects of acute and chronic right ventricular pacing had also been increasing in the literature.[5] Therefore, the author proceeded with HBP and AV nodal ablation proximal to the site of His pacing, which resulted in preservation of intrinsic activation with excellent rate control and rapid improvement in the patient's condition.

This result was replicated in the author's first case series of patients with longstanding AF and dilated cardiomyopathy in whom HBP was shown to be feasible and was associated with improvements in left ventricular dimensions and function.[6]

HISTORY: ANATOMY AND ELECTROPHYSIOLOGY OF THE HIS BUNDLE

Although the adverse hemodynamic impact of right ventricular apical pacing had been demonstrated as early as 1925 by Carl Wiggers, several scientific and technologic advancements were required to enable the widespread use of permanent HBP.[7] Because early transvenous leads were secured with passive fixation tines and predominantly implanted by surgeons, the right ventricular apex became the default site for permanent pacemakers. Only with the advent of active fixation screw in leads could anatomic or electrophysiologic lead localization become a consideration.

The anatomy of the His bundle was first described by William His in 1893. A subsequent monography in 1906 by Sunao Tawara gave a more extensive anatomic and histologic description of the His Purkinje network and first dubbed the term "conduction system."[8] It was only in 1969 that Scherlag and colleagues[9] described intravascular catheter recordings of the His bundle in humans. Soon after, Scherlag and colleagues[10,11] demonstrated temporary transvenous HBP in humans and subsequently stable

Cardiac and Vascular Center, Arrhythmia Center, Robert Packer Hospital, 1 Guthrie Square, Sayre, PA 18840, USA
E-mail address: prmode@yahoo.com

Card Electrophysiol Clin 10 (2018) 453–459
https://doi.org/10.1016/j.ccep.2018.05.007

models of transcatheter HBP were developed in canines. Importantly, these studies outlined a strategy of using stabilized recording catheters to provide a fluoroscopic landmark for the His bundle during lead placement.

The author's initial experience in early 1995 was done by defining the His bundle with a femoral mapping catheter as a target for a stylet-driven lead.[6,11] Given the known anatomy of the His bundle, a J-shaped stylet was modified to include a second curve orthogonal to the plane of the "J" in order to position the screw in line with the long axis of the His bundle.[8] Later, the development of preformed and steerable "His bundle sheaths" significantly improved lead stability during delivery and several investigators have demonstrated procedural success by using the pacing lead as a mapping catheter.[12–14] However, the use of a dedicated mapping catheter and even three-dimensional mapping may be of value with procedural inexperience, complex anatomy, or in the setting of AV nodal ablation.[15,16]

Once localized, the final challenge in achieving His bundle lead placement is achieving fixation in the fibrous sheath surrounding the bundle within the membranous septum.[17] In the author's initial experience with a 1.5 mm screw-in helix, dislodgement during implant was common and it was observed that a slight advancement of the His lead into the septum often yielded a significantly lower pacing threshold than achieved by the mapping catheter.[6] Based on this experience, a Medtronic-sponsored single-center investigational device exemption study using a custom 1.8 mm screw in lead model 10514 was conducted. The later use of a longer 1.8 mm helix of the Medtronic 3830 lead (Minneapolis, Minnesota) likely improves procedural success and chronic capture thresholds.[12–14]

Based on the electrophysiologic properties of the His bundle and studies by Scherlag and colleagues,[6,10,18] the criteria for "direct" or "selective" HBP were developed:

1. Concordance of the paced and native QRS and T wave complexes on 12-lead electrocardiogram
2. Equivalent pace-ventricular and His-ventricular intervals

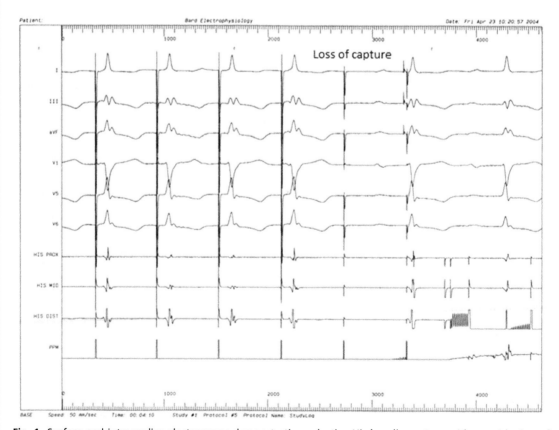

Fig. 1. Surface and intracardiac electrograms demonstrating selective His bundle capture with no widening of the paced QRS and abrupt loss of capture with decreasing stimulus voltage.

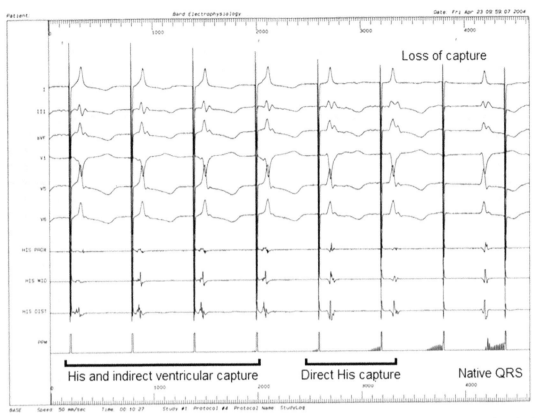

Fig. 2. Indirect ventricular capture by His bundle lead at high output. As the pacing stimulus is reduced from high output, the widened QRS with ventricular and His bundle capture (beats 1–4) transitions to a narrow QRS equivalent to the native QRS (direct His capture in beats 5 and 6), and at even lower pacing thresholds there is complete loss of capture (stimulus 7).

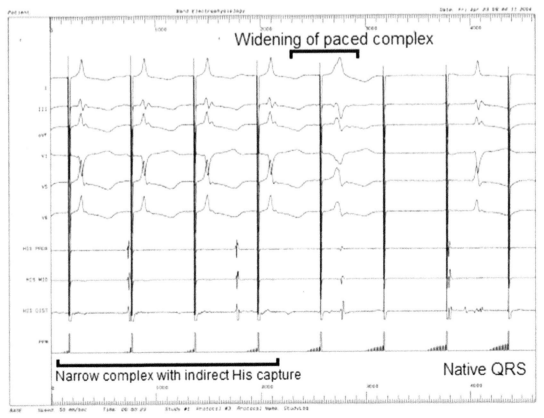

Fig. 3. Indirect His capture does not demonstrate a single capture threshold.

3. All-or-none capture as demonstrated by the absence of QRS widening, with sequentially lower pacing output with abrupt loss of capture (**Fig. 1**)

Several important observations informed these criteria:

- With high pacing thresholds, a lead that selectively captures the His bundle can indirectly capture the ventricle or atria (**Fig. 2**)
- Indirect or nonselective capture of the His bundle can lead to a narrow QRS, which is not equivalent to the native QRS. Decreasing the pacing stimulus at such sites demonstrates that they do not satisfy the third criteria (**Fig. 3**)
- In patients with His Purkinje disease, HBP can induce cardiac resynchronization (**Fig. 4**)[19]

These criteria were later validated by other investigators and expanded to define selective and nonselective His capture in patients with both intact and diseased His Purkinje conduction (**Table 1**).[20,21]

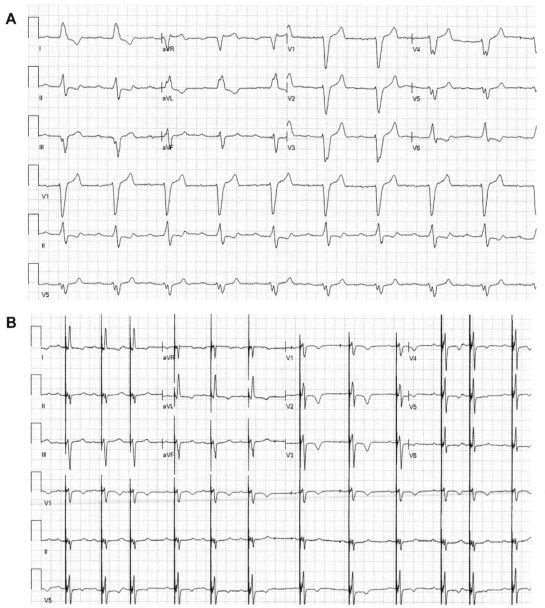

Fig. 4. Narrowing of QRS by His bundle pacing. (*A*) Native QRS with left bundle branch block. (*B*) Reversal of left bundle branch block with His bundle pacing.

Table 1
Definitions of selective and nonselective His bundle pacing from a multicenter His Bundle pacing collaborative working group

Baseline		His Purkinje Disease	
Response to Pacing	Normal QRS	With QRS Narrowing	Without QRS Narrowing
Selective HBP Criteria	• S-QRS = H-QRS with isoelectric interval • Discrete local ventricular electrogram in HBP lead with S-V = H-V • Paced QRS = native QRS • Single capture threshold (all or none capture)	• S-QRS ≤ H-QRS with isoelectric interval • Discrete local ventricular electrogram in HBP lead • Paced QRS < native QRS • 2 distinct capture thresholds (HBP with BBB correction, HBP without BBB correction)	• H-QRS with isoelectric interval • Discrete local ventricular electrogram in HBP lead • Paced QRS = native QRS • Single capture threshold (HBP with BBB)

Adapted from Cantù F, De Filippo P, Cardano P, et al. Validation of criteria for selective his bundle and para-hisian permanent pacing. Pacing Clin Electrophysiol 2006;29(12):1326–33; with permission.

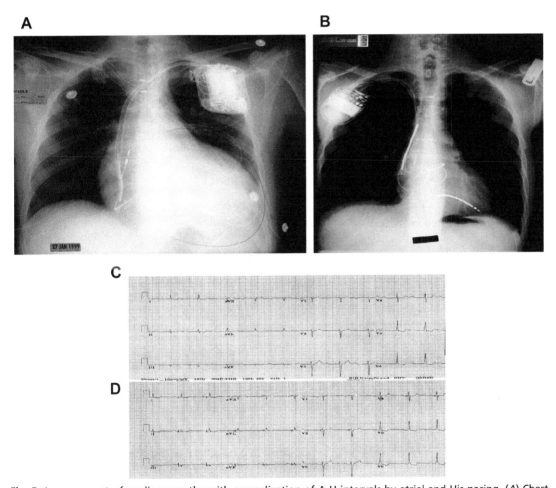

Fig. 5. Improvement of cardiomyopathy with normalization of A-H intervals by atrial and His pacing. (*A*) Chest radiograph from implant in 1999. (*B*) Chest radiograph at follow-up in 2004 after reimplant on the right side of lead fracture. (*C*) Patient's baseline electrocardiogram demonstrating atrioventricular nodal disease. (*D*) His paced electrocardiogram demonstrating normalization of the PR interval and maintenance of a narrow native QRS.

HBP IN HEART FAILURE: RESTORING INTRAVENTRICULAR AND ATRIOVENTRICULAR SYNCHRONY

Since the author's initial experience, several clinical situations in patients with heart failure in which HBP can be applied have been investigated.

1. *Resynchronization with HBP:* the potential for HBP to induce cardiac resynchronization had been noted in the studies by Sherlag and colleagues[22] and attributed this effect to preselection of bundle branch fibers. Reversal of left bundle branch block when pacing slightly distally and with higher output was also identified.[19] This effect has since been replicated in clinical studies by several investigators.[23–25] Importantly, Lustgarten and colleagues[26] have demonstrated similar echocardiographic and functional status improvements with resynchronization by HBP in comparison with biventricular pacing in a blinded crossover trial.

2. *HPB in patients with AF and Heart Failure:* subsequent to the author's initial experience, a larger series of 59 patients with heart failure and AF who underwent His bundle pacing and AV nodal ablation at the 2012 Dead Sea Symposium was reported.[27] In this cohort, rate and rhythm control with AV nodal ablation and HBP was associated with improved functional status and ejection fraction. Recently, this strategy of His bundle pacing and ablation for AF was validated by Huang and colleagues[28] in patients with heart failure and both reduced and preserved ejection fraction.

Restoring Intraventricular and Atrioventricular Synchrony

Where His pacing was associated with a narrower QRS than biventricular pacing, the author's group had initiated a crossover study between HBP and biventricular pacing.[29] However, the protocol was terminated due to patient's (blinded) preference for HBP and early rehospitalization in the biventricular pacing group. Importantly, Lustgarten and colleagues[26] have demonstrated similar echocardiographic and functional status improvements with resynchronization by HBP in comparison with biventricular pacing in a blinded crossover trial.

In addition to maintenance or restoration of intraventricular synchrony, HBP has the potential to optimize AV synchrony and the contribution of the atria to cardiac output. In a small series of patients with heart failure and AV nodal disease, the author saw dramatic improvements in cardiac

geometry, ejection fraction, and functional capacity after implantation of atrial, His, and right ventricular leads (**Fig. 5**).[30] Sohaib and colleagues[31] have demonstrated that HBP is also comparable to biventricular pacing in patients for optimization of AV delays. In a cohort of 16 patients with heart failure and PR prolongation without left bundle branch block, they showed that HBP and biventricular pacing resulted in similar augmentation of systolic blood pressure compared with native conduction, by a magnitude (~4 mm Hg) comparable to that seen in larger studies such as PATH-CHF.[31,32] Larger and longer-term studies evaluating HBP as an alternative to biventricular pacing are ongoing and discussed in Harsimran Saini and colleagues' article, "Future Developments in His Bundle Pacing," in this issue.

SUMMARY

In summary, a century of advancements in anatomy, physiology, and technology have made HBP a feasible and potentially optimal site of permanent pacing. The electrophysiology of the His bundle implies precise criteria that can be used to define selective HBP. By using the native conduction system, HBP is versatile and can be used not only for brady indications but also as a means of rate control in AF, cardiac resynchronization, and AV optimization.

REFERENCES

1. Deshmukh P, Anderson K. Direct His bundle pacing: novel approach to permanent pacing in patients with severe left ventricular dysfunction and atrial fibrillation [abstract]. Pacing Clin Electrophysiol 1996;19(4):644–743.
2. Packer DL, Bardy GH, Worley SJ, et al. Tachycardia-induced cardiomyopathy: a reversible form of left ventricular dysfunction. Am J Cardiol 1986;57(8): 563–70.
3. Cruz FE, Cheriex EC, Smeets JL, et al. Reversibility of tachycardia-induced cardiomyopathy after cure of incessant supraventricular tachycardia. J Am Coll Cardiol 1990;16(3):739–44.
4. Kay GN, Bubien RS, Epstein AE, et al. Effect of catheter ablation of the atrioventricular junction on quality of life and exercise tolerance in paroxysmal atrial fibrillation. Am J Cardiol 1988;62(10 Pt 1):741–4.
5. Badke FR, Boinay P, Covell JW. Effects of ventricular pacing on regional left ventricular performance in the dog. Am J Physiol 1980;238(6): H858–67.
6. Deshmukh P, Casavant DA, Romanyshyn M, et al. Permanent, direct His-bundle pacing: a novel approach to cardiac pacing in patients with normal

His-Purkinje activation. Circulation 2000;101(8): 869–77.

7. Wiggers CJ. The muscular reactions of the mammalian ventricles to artificial surface stimuli. Am J Physiol 1925;73(2):346–78.

8. Tawara S. Das Reizleitungssystem Des Säugetierherzens [The Conduction System of the Mammalian Heart]. Jena: Gustav Fischer; 1906. Suma K, Shimada M, trans. London, UK: Imperial College Press; 2000.

9. Scherlag BJ, Lau SH, Helfant RH, et al. Catheter technique for recording His bundle activity in man. Circulation 1969;39(1):13–8.

10. Narula OS, Scherlag BJ, Samet P. Pervenous pacing of the specialized conducting system in man: His bundle and A-V nodal stimulation. Circulation 1970;41(1):77–87.

11. Mabo P, Scherlag BJ, Munsif A, et al. A technique for stable His-bundle recording and pacing: electrophysiological and hemodynamic correlates. Pacing Clin Electrophysiol 1995;18(10):1894–901.

12. Zanon F, Baracca E, Aggio S, et al. A feasible approach for direct His-bundle pacing using a new steerable catheter to facilitate precise lead placement. J Cardiovasc Electrophysiol 2006;17(1):29–33.

13. Dandamudi G, Vijayaraman P. How to perform permanent His bundle pacing in routine clinical practice. Heart Rhythm 2016;13(6):1362–6.

14. Lustgarten D. Step-wise approach to permanent His bundle pacing. J Innovation Card Rhythm Management 2016;7(4):2313–21.

15. Ringwala S, Knight BP, Verma N. Permanent His-bundle pacing at the time of atrioventricular node ablation: a three-dimensional mapping approach. HeartRhythm Case Rep 2017. https://doi.org/10.1016/j.hrcr.2017.04.005.

16. Kean AC, Kay WA, Patel JK, et al. Permanent nonselective His bundle pacing in an adult with L-transposition of the great arteries and complete AV block. Pacing Clin Electrophysiol 2017;40(11):1313–7.

17. Kurosawa H, Becker A. The conduction bundle at the atrioventricular junction an anatomical study. Eur J Cardiothorac Surg 1989;3(4):283–7.

18. Williams DO, Scherlag BJ, Hope RR, et al. Selective versus non-selective His bundle pacing. Cardiovasc Res 1976;10(1):91–100.

19. Deshmukh PM, Romanyshyn M. Direct His-bundle pacing: present and future. Pacing Clin Electrophysiol 2004;27(6 Pt 2):862–70.

20. Cantù F, De Filippo P, Cardano P, et al. Validation of criteria for selective his bundle and para-hisian permanent pacing. Pacing Clin Electrophysiol 2006; 29(12):1326–33.

21. Vijayaraman P, Dandamudi G, Zanon F, et al. Permanent His bundle pacing: recommendations from a multicenter His bundle pacing collaborative working group for standardization of definitions, implant measurements, and follow-up. Heart Rhythm 2018; 15(3):460–8.

22. El-Sherif N, Amay-Y-Leon F, Schonfield C, et al. Normalization of bundle branch block patterns by distal His bundle pacing. Clinical and experimental evidence of longitudinal dissociation in the pathologic his bundle. Circulation 1978;57(3):473–83.

23. Lustgarten DL, Calame S, Crespo EM, et al. Electrical resynchronization induced by direct His-bundle pacing. Heart Rhythm 2010;7(1):15–21.

24. Ajijola OA, Upadhyay GA, Macias C, et al. Permanent His-bundle pacing for cardiac resynchronization therapy: initial feasibility study in lieu of left ventricular lead. Heart Rhythm 2017;14(9):1353–61.

25. Sharma PS, Dandamudi G, Herweg B, et al. Permanent His-bundle pacing as an alternative to biventricular pacing for cardiac resynchronization therapy: a multicenter experience. Heart Rhythm 2018;15(3):413–20.

26. Lustgarten DL, Crespo EM, Arkhipova-Jenkins I, et al. His-bundle pacing versus biventricular pacing in cardiac resynchronization therapy patients: a crossover design comparison. Heart Rhythm 2015; 12(7):1548–57.

27. Deshmukh P, Deshmukh A, Anderson K, et al. Direct His bundle pacing and atrioventricular nodal ablation: an alernatie to achieving "rhythm control". Oral presentation, 11th Dead Sea Symposium. Jerusalem (Israel): February 26, 2012.

28. Huang W, Su L, Wu S, et al. Benefits of permanent His bundle pacing combined with atrioventricular node ablation in atrial fibrillation patients with heart failure with both preserved and reduced left ventricular ejection fraction. J Am Heart Assoc 2017;6(4) [pii:e005309].

29. Deshmukh P, Padmanabhan S, Sattur S, et al. Comparison of direct His bundle and biventricular pacing. Heart Rhythm 2009;6(5):S375.

30. Deshmukh P, Deshmukh A, Romanyshyn M, et al. Direct His bundle triple site pacing: a novel alternative to biventricular pacing. Heart Rhythm 2009;6(5): S1–54.

31. Sohaib SMA, Wright I, Lim E, et al. Atrioventricular optimized direct His bundle pacing improves acute hemodynamic function in patients with heart failure and pr interval prolongation without left bundle branch block. JACC Clin Electrophysiol 2015;1(6): 582–91.

32. Auricchio A, Stellbrink C, Block M, et al. Effect of pacing chamber and atrioventricular delay on acute systolic function of paced patients with congestive heart failure. Circulation 1999;99(23):2993–3001.

His Bundle (Conduction System) Pacing
A Contemporary Appraisal

Alan Sugrue, MBChB[a], Subir Bhatia, MD[b],
Vaibhav R. Vaidya, MBBS[a], Ugur Kucuk, MD[a],
Siva K. Mulpuru, MD[a], Samuel J. Asirvatham, MD[a],*

KEYWORDS

- His bundle • His bundle pacing • Cardiac resynchronization therapy

KEY POINTS

- Conduction system pacing offers an attractive approach to achieving physiologic pacing in those who those who require a ventricular lead.
- Benefits reported include improvement in left, with improvement in left ventricular ejection fraction, functional status, heart failure hospitalizations, and possibly mortality.
- Apart from technical aspects of the procedure, lead outcomes (in particular lead thresholds and lead stability) represent one of the leading barriers to current everyday application.

INTRODUCTION

The transformation and evolution of pacemakers over the past 70 years is remarkable, from the classic indication in the 1950s of complete heart block with Stoke-Adams seizures to today's practice with a sprawling number of indications. Many of the first descriptions of pacemakers were preceded by the word, *artificial*, and, they were true to that term, because asynchronous pacing was the initial modality and was not representative of typical physiologic conduction. Even the earliest pioneers of cardiac pacing recognized this and desired a means of achieving and producing more physiologic pacing—a goal unachievable at the time due to both knowledge and technological limitations. Although the development of synchronous pacing (first implanted in humans in 1962[1]) was a breakthrough, it was always recognized that this was not natural physiologic pacing with reliance on the right ventricular (RV) apex for placement due to ease of access and lead stability.

As data propagated the potential adverse effects of nonphysiologic chronic RV pacing,[2–8] there was innovative growth in pacing modes and lead delivery technology, causing a shift away from the apex in search of new pacing sites. Initial studies focused on the RV outflow tract but subsequent equivocal studies[9,10] saw hesitation with routine use in clinical practice. The His bundle (HB) emerged as an alluring physiologic target, and although initially considered in the 1980s, it was not until the 2000s that it gathered steam. Of all the possible pacing sites, it was considered by far the most physiologic form of pacing with use of the native conduction systems to enable native activation of the ventricles. Since Deshmukh and

Disclosures: S.J. Asirvatham receives no significant honoraria and is a consultant with Abiomed, Aegis, ATP, Atricure, Biotronik, Boston Scientific, FocusStart, Medtronic, Medtelligence, Nevro, Sanovas, Sorin Medical, Spectranetics, St. Jude, Sanofi-Aventis, Wolters Kluwer, Elsevier, and Zoll. All other authors have no disclosures.
[a] Division of Heart Rhythm, Department of Cardiovascular Diseases, Mayo Clinic, 200 1st Street South West, Rochester, MN 55902, USA; [b] Division of Internal Medicine, Department of Medicine, Mayo Clinic, 200 1st Street South West, Rochester, MN 55902, USA
* Corresponding author. Department of Cardiovascular Diseases, Mayo Clinic Rochester, 200 1st Street Southwest, Rochester, MN 55905.
E-mail address: asirvatham.samuel@mayo.edu

colleagues' seminal article in 2000,[11] the growth and interest in HB pacing (HBP) has been slow but exponential, especially within the past 2 years (**Fig. 1**).

There is much confusion in the literature regarding HBP, with inconsistently used terminology and inexact appreciation of the precise portion of the anatomic conduction system stimulated. We, therefore, prefer to use the term, *conduction system pacing* (CSP),[12] which refers to the pacing of the conduction system to reproduce a normal QRS morphology. When this occurs without surrounding ventricular myocardial capture, we suggest the term, *selective CSP* (SCSP). We prefer these terms because the close association of the conduction tissues in this HB area makes it difficult at times to appreciate the exact stimulated structure (HB, atrioventricular [AV] node, distal AV node transitional zone, and proximal branches). Furthermore, the resultant activation is dependent on the pacing output, electrode dimension, type, and orientation relative to the conduction tissue and myocardium.

This review aims to provide insight into the historical growth of HBP (SCSP) and provide a contemporary appraisal. The unique anatomy and physiology of the conduction system in both normal and abnormal hearts, current tools and techniques for lead implantation, current outcomes, and thoughts on future directions are examined.

A BRIEF HISTORY OF THE HIS BUNDLE

The first description of the HB dates back to 1893 when Wilhelm His, Jr, described an embryogenic muscle that united the right auricle and ventricles.[13] He stated, "After long search I have succeeded in finding a muscle bundle which unites the auricular and ventricular septal walls, and which, up to now, has escaped observation because of incomplete exposure, for it is visible in its entire extent only when the septa are cut exactly in their longitudinal direction." It was not until 1958, however, that the HB recordings were made by Alanis and colleagues[14] (**Fig. 2**), who studied these signals in animals. The first recordings made in a human were in 1959 and subsequently with intravascular catheters in 1960. Although the potential clinical utility of recruiting the HB at this time was understood, research remained quiescent until the year 2000.[11]

ANATOMY
Normal Heart

The HB is a continuation of the distal part of the AV node, measuring up to 20 mm in length and 4 mm in diameter. It is composed of mostly large Purkinje-type cells, which are longitudinally oriented. The proximal cells of the penetrating portion are heterogeneous and resemble the cells of the compact node; the distal cells of the HB are similar to the proximal bundle branch cells. The anterior and posterior descending coronary arteries provide a dual blood supply to the HB, making it less prone to ischemic damage. The HB is innervated by both adrenergic and cholinergic nerve fibers. The density of innervation to the HB is higher than that found in the ventricular myocardium.

The boundary of the AV node and HB has not been clearly defined anatomically. Histologically, it is the point at which the cell type becomes predominately of the large Purkinje type and at which most of the cells become oriented parallel in a longitudinal direction and cease interweaving. This longitudinal division of the HB by collagen is a distinct histologic difference from the AV node.[15] Toward the lower end of the bundle, the fibers become progressively larger, which tends to produce faster conduction velocity. Anatomically, the AV-HB junction usually occurs at the point at which the HB penetrates the central fibrous body and leaves the AV node (**Fig. 3**).[15] The HB passes through the fibrous core of the central fibrinous body in a leftward direction towards the ventricular septum and then continues through the annulus fibrosis before penetrating the membranous septum for 1 cm to 2 cm before finally dividing into the left and right bundle branches. The HB course is anatomically divided into 3 portions: (1) nonpenetrating (as it passes through the annulus fibrosis), (2) penetrating (within the fibrinous tissue of the central body and membranous septum), and (3) branching portion (bifurcation into the left and right bundle branches at the crest of the muscular ventricular septum).

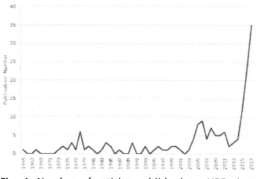

Fig. 1. Number of articles published on HBP since 1965.

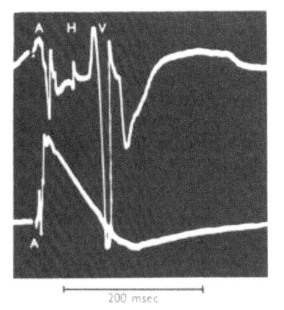

Fig. 2. First recording of the HB signal in animals.

Ventricular Septal Defect

In ventricular septal defects (VSDs), the HB runs along the inferior posterior rim of the VSD and tends to be more elongated and generally on the left ventricular side. When surgical closure of a VSD is attempted, to avoid complications of HB disruption, it is vital when suturing the right septal surface that the sutures are at least 2 mm away from the rim of the ventricular septum. Generally, this HB electrogram is recorded as expected along the superior-medial rim of the tricuspid valve.

Atrioventricular Septal Defects

The HB penetrates the apex of the nodal triangle (anterior to the coronary sinus ostium, posterior insertion of the bridging tendon to the posterior fibrous area, and posterior bridge leaflet) and runs along the lower rim of the ventricular septum, resulting in a posteriorly displaced conduction network. Accordingly, the HB electrogram is recorded along the right side of the AV defect lower than expected and in the setting of patches or repair this signal may be attenuated.

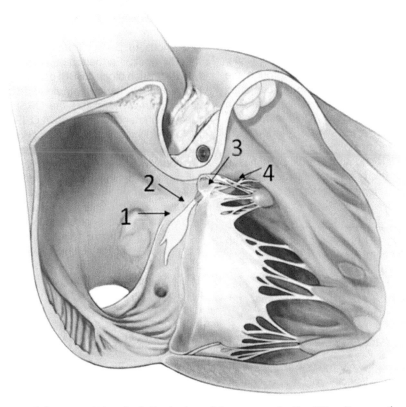

Fig. 3. Anatomy of the HB. 1, AV node. 2, Beginning of the nonpenetrating HB as it passes through the annulus fibrosis. 3, The His penetrating the central fibrosis body. 4, Just after the branching portion of the HB.

Tetralogy of Fallot

In tetralogy of Fallot, the position of the AV node is normal as the HB passes close to the crest of the interventricular septum and may pass slightly to the left of the inferior margin of the VSD. The presence of an extended ventriculo-infundibular fold largely determines the proximity of the bundle to the crest of the inferior VSD. If the ventriculo-infundibular fold is well developed, it may form a continuous muscle border in combination with the posterior limb of the trabecular septomarginalis, thus creating a separation of the tricuspid annulus from the VSD covering the membranous septum. In most cases in which there is a malalignment of VSD, the HB runs on the posterior and inferior rim to the defect, allowing a VSD closure without injury to the HB.[16]

Transposition of the Great Arteries

In dextroposition of the great arteries, the conduction system is normally positioned. Distortion of the atrial anatomy post–atrial switch can make it challenging, however, to obtain an HB electrogram, and for a more precise HB recording, a retroaortic approach is usually necessary.

In congenitally corrected transposition of the great arteries, the conduction system anatomy is abnormal. The AV node usually has 2 aspects (anterior and posterior) leading to anterior and posterior HB. The posterior node (usually normally positioned in the triangle of Koch) is hypoplastic. The HB is elongated and infiltrates through the fibrous trigone and continues along the cephalad margin of the outflow tract in the subendocardium of the ventricular myocardium. On reaching the ventricular septum, the HB moves inferiorly and then descend anterior along the septum before giving rise to the left and right bundle branches. If a VSD is present, this is a situation where the HB may travel superior along the upper rim of the VSD.

Ebstein Anomaly

The AV node and HB are similar in hearts with Ebstein anomaly compared with normal hearts. In approximately 90% of patients with Ebstein anomaly, however, the entry of the HB occurs before the apex of the triangle of Koch is reached, and its length is usually shorter.

HIS BUNDLE PHYSIOLOGY

The electrical signal travels through the AV node with a conduction velocity of approximately 0.05 m/s. On reaching the HB, there is an abrupt increase in speed to approximately 1.5 m/s (range 1.3–1.7 m/s), where it then moves through the bundles to the ventricular myocardium. In a healthy heart, the time of onset of HB depolarization to ventricular myocardial electrogram is approximately 35 milliseconds (ms) to 55 ms (H–V interval). The earliest area of ventricular muscle activation on the left side is midseptal (27 ms ± 2 ms), and this is matched by midseptal activation on the right side at the junction of the right bundle branch and the base of the anterior papillary (27 ms ± 3 ms).[17] Neither sympathetic nor vagal stimulation effects normal conduction in the HB. Unlike the AV node, the electric activity of the HB can be recorded with a catheter and typically this signal is a sharp spike 10 ms to 25 ms in duration interposed between a local atrial and ventricular signal. The HB can be recorded from both the left side and right side of the heart. On the left side, this is at the junction of the noncoronary cusp and the right coronary cusp under the aortic valve. Noninvasive recording of the HB is not currently available, although methods to do this have been proposed,[18] with a recent focus on microwavelet analysis during the surface ECG PR interval.[19]

Normalization of the QRS

As discussed previously, the HB is an alluring target because it can enable normal physiologic conduction, negating the potentially harmful consequences of pacing from other sites, such as the RV apex. Furthermore, in patients with left bundle branch block (LBBB) or right bundle branch block (RBBB), it can restore electrical synchronization (narrow/normalize the QRS) (**Fig. 4**). The reestablishment of a narrow QRS complex by SCSP (HBP) represents an intact His-Purkinje system or the capability of overcoming impaired conduction within the His-Purkinje system. The mechanism behind electrical synchronization in CSP is likely an amalgamation of 3 mechanisms: longitudinal dissociation, source-sink mismatch, and virtual electrode polarization effect.

Predestined fibers or longitudinal dissociation is a proposed concept in which fibers within the HB are predestined for the left and right bundles. This concept was first proposed by Kaufman and Rothberger in 1919,[20] with the anatomic basis for this theory described in human and canine hearts in the 1970s by James and Sherf.[15] In this study, they reported that one of the more striking histologic features of the HB was the partitioning of the fibers by collagen. This collagen was longitudinally orientated and several millimeters in length. Additionally, they noted that there were occasionally crossover connections between the bundles (transverse connections). Narula[21] was the first to

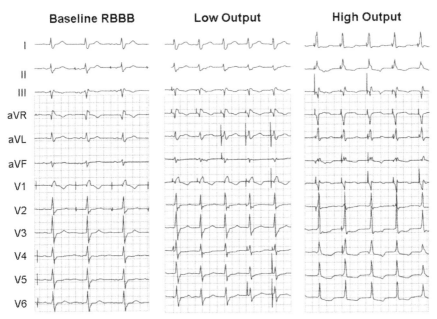

Fig. 4. Narrowing of QRS by CSP. Baseline ECG shows an RBBB (left panel), which does not resolve with low output pacing (middle panel). At higher outputs (right panel) the QRS narrows and represents more physiologic.

demonstrate the clinical significance of longitudinal dissociation. In patients with LBBB or isolated left axis deviation by stimulation of different portions of the HB, the baseline ECG pattern could be abolished, resulting in normalization of QRS duration or axis. This observation was believed to be due to longitudinal dissociation, because stimulation of the HB proximal to the proposed intra-His lesion would result in ventricular depolarization similar to normal sinus rhythm, but HB stimulation distal to the lesion could result in narrow QRS complexes due to synchronous impulse conduction to both the bundle branches (**Fig. 5**).

Sherif and collegaeus[22] and Puech and colleagues[23] provided further experimental evidence of longitudinal dissociation. More recently Barba-Pichardo and colleagues[24] and other investigators[25–29] showed that QRS normalization was possible and reported to be successful approximately 75% of the time. Although there is significant evidence supporting longitudinal dissociation, it must also be noted that the view of predestined fibers has been challenged in the past.[30,31] In particular, Lazzara and colleagues[32] examined explicitly the functional role of the transverse fibers observed by James and Sherf and showed that a small residual of intact right bundle after an incision could activate the whole bundle distal to the incision with undetectable alterations in the distal activation pattern (**Fig. 6**). An incision in the left bundle branch could occasionally result in alterations of a few milliseconds in the activation sequence if there was a significant

lesion. Furthermore, from microelectrode exploration, it was established that distal activation of the incised fibers a few millimeters from the incision occurred antegrade and transversely from intact residual HB interconnections.

The longitudinal dissociation theory also fails to address adequately the observation that HPB can overcome disease more distal than the HB/branch junctions, suggesting there are other mechanisms at play. Part of this could be explained by source-sink mismatch.[28,33] In many patients with distal His-Purkinje disease, there is usually some element of proximal disease present, signifying that there is a decrease in the number of conducting cells proximally (source), which are available to produce a sufficient voltage gradient to depolarize through the diseased distal His-Purkinje system (sink). Thus, increased source power can lead to depolarization of the diseased tissue. An additional theory proposed is that of virtual electrode polarization. This is an electrical phenomenon by which an electric stimulus creates regions of depolarization and hyperpolarization, which can cause excitation of previously refractory tissue and thereby provide a pathway for propagation.[34,35]

SELECTIVE CONDUCTION SYSTEM PACING: TOOLS AND TECHNIQUES
Tools

Tools and techniques for CSP have evolved from the original description with application of stimulation electrodes onto the surface of the atrial

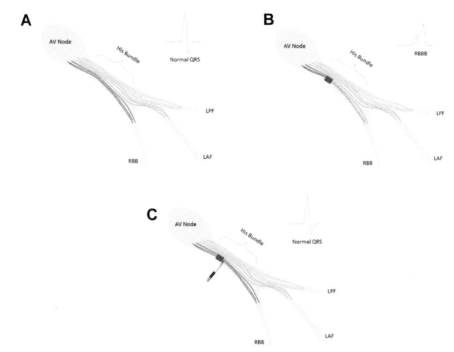

Fig. 5. Longitudinal dissociation theory showing predestined fibers. (*A*) Normal His-Purkinje system activation. (*B*) His-Purkinje system activation in the setting of RBBB. (*C*) Pacing distal to the site of block leading to normal His-Purkinje system activation. AV Node, Atrioventricular Node; LAF, left anterior fascicle; LPF, left posterior fascicle; RBB, Right bundle branch.

endocardium close to the ventricle.[36] Scherlag and colleagues[37] performed the first localized HBP using a plunge wire method, which was followed by Narula and colleagues,[38] who temporarily paced the HB percutaneously using a bipolar electrode catheter connected to an external

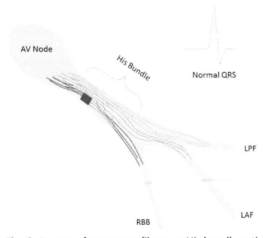

Fig. 6. Impact of transverse fibers on His bundle activation. It is proposed that these transverse fibers can overcome a block proximal and enable relatively normal HB activation. AV Node, Atrioventricular Node; LAF, left anterior fascicle; LPF, left posterior fascicle; RBB, Right bundle branch.

pacemaker, with a stimulus strength of 15 mA (with an assumed HB resistance of 500, equivalent to approximately 7.5 V). An approach to permanent pacing (specifically septal His-Purkinje pacing) was not described until 1992,[39] when an active fixation helical screw composed of platinum-iridium, 4.5 mm in length, was inserted through an introducer placed through the right atrial appendage in a canine model. In 1999, Amitani and colleagues[40] in animal studies proposed a method for permanent HPB by using a screw in lead with an 11F guide catheter to help with anchoring. Two types of screw-in leads were tested: Medtronic 4068 (Medtronic, Minneapolis, Minnesota) and 4 bipolar leads of Intermedics (Freeport, Texas). The first human studies were reported by Deskmukh and colleagues in 1996[41] and then published in 2000.[11] In these studies, a Medtronic bipolar screw-in lead (sweet tip 4145) and a modified J-shaped stylet with a secondary distal curve allowed the lead to be correctly oriented. In 2006, Zanon and colleagues[42] published on the use of the steerable catheter and showed a potential increase in the success of implantation with a steerable catheter used to deliver the screw-in lead. Lastly, Vazquez, Barba-Pichardo and colleague[43–45] used active fixation Tendril models (St. Jude Medical, Minneapolis, Minnesota).

Despite different devices and tools being historically used, at present, only Medtronic offers a specialized lead and the delivery tool necessary for HBP (CSP) (**Fig. 7**). The deflectable catheter most commonly used is a Medtronic C315 His nondeflectable sheath, which has a 7F outer diameter and 5.4F inner diameter. The C315 has both a proximal curve toward the tricuspid valve annulus and a second curve toward the septum that delivers the lead perpendicular to the septum to enable superior fixation. A C304 deflectable sheath (9F) is an alternative. It can be challenging, however, to secure the lead in the His location with this sheath. The delivery sheaths for CSP are designed for left pectoral implantation, but right-sided implant can be performed. The lead used most commonly today is an active fixation screw (SelectSecure 3830, Medtronic), which is 4.1F in diameter, has no inner lumen, and has an exposed screw of length 1.8 mm. The distal electrode screw is steroid eluting to allow for improved pacing thresholds.

Conduction System Pacing: Defining Key Terminology

Regarding nomenclature, as discussed previously, we prefer the term, CSP. The concept of selective versus nonselective pacing was first described by Williams and colleagues in 1976[46] and is an important concept to understand. Broadly there are 2 forms of conduction system capture: selective, in which the pacing stimulus purely captures the conduction system, and nonselective, in which there is fusion capture of the conduction system and adjacent ventricular myocardium. There has been a lack of consistency in the literature in

HBP, and, consequently, a working group was formed and recently published criteria and definitions.[47] The authors agree with these definitions, with the addition of changing HBP for CSP.

SCSP (**Fig. 8**) is defined as follows:

1. Pacing stimulus to QRS onset equal to native His-QRS onset interval
2. The local ventricular electrogram separate from the pacing artifact
3. Electrocardiographic concordance of QRS and T-wave complexes, similar to baseline
4. Single capture threshold observed

CSP is defined as follows:

1. No isoelectric interval between pacing stimulus and QRS complex
2. The local ventricular electrogram pulled close to the pacing stimulus due to local myocardial capture and therefore not seen as a discrete component
3. The electrical axis of the paced QRS complex must be concordant with the electrical axis of the spontaneous QRS (if known)
4. Narrowing of the QRS complex at higher output due to fusion between the RV and His-bundle capture and widening of the QRS complex at lower output due to loss of His-bundle capture or vice versa

It is unclear at this stage which is better. SCSP preserves physiologic repolarization and intrinsic ST and T–wave patterns and consequently may be favored. Whether SCSP results in greater clinical benefit compared with non-selective conduction system pacing (NSCSP), however, remains unclear. This will be important

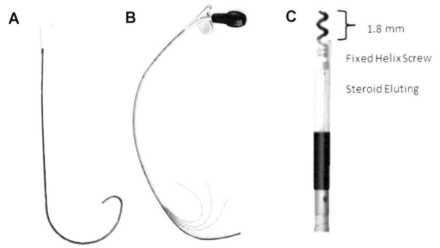

Fig. 7. (*A*) C315 His nondeflectable sheath. (*B*) A C304 deflectable sheath. (*C*) SelectSecure 3830. (*Courtesy of* Medtronic Inc, Minneapolis, MN; with permission.)

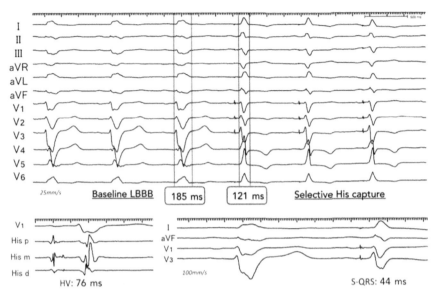

Fig. 8. Selective HBP. There is clear narrowing of the QRS as well as clear separating of the ventricular electrogram from the pacing artifact. (*Data from* Ajijola O, Upadhyay GA, Macias C, et al. Permanent His-bundle pacing for cardiac resynchronization therapy: initial feasibility study in lieu of left ventricular lead. Heart Rhythm 2017;14(9):1353–61.)

to address in future studies because of the potential threshold and R-wave sensing advantages of nonselective CSP.

Technique of Implantation

From the outset, there is a significant learning curve with CSP placement, with a mean number of lead positioning attempts reported to be approximately 4. After obtaining venous access and insertion of a sheath (preferably with a short 7F peel-away sheath), a wire is placed into the right atrium, on which the Select-Secure sheath is placed. When the wire is retracted, the sheath assumes a septal orientation. The lead is then put through the delivery sheath. The lead, as discussed previously, is lumen-less, and only the distal electrode is exposed. Electrograms are then recorded in a unipolar fashion, with the HB mapped by clocking or counter-clocking the sheath and by pulling or pushing the lead. Once the HB is recorded, the lead is screwed by tuning 5 to 8 clockwise turns. A current of injury observed may be predictive of a good response and threshold. The sheath is then pulled back and slack created on the lead. Threshold testing is usually performed at 1.0-ms pulse width. When values are satisfactory, the lead is secured with a suture sleeve. The lead is then connected to the pulse generator.

APPRAISAL OF CURRENT DATA
What Is Known and What the Issues Are

Patient demographics
To date, most of the published data on CSP have focused on patients with AV nodal disease (including patients after AV node ablation, which was the focus of many early studies), patients with infranodal disease, and, more recently, as a means to provide cardiac resynchronization therapy (CRT) (**Table 1**). Across all studies, there is a trend towards more implants in men. It is unclear if gender or age plays a role in outcomes, as has been observed in CRT therapy with a left ventricular lead,[48,49] and this should be examined in future studies.

Conduction system sensing
With CSP, there is limited ventricular myocardium, and, consequently, the sensed R waves are often smaller than those recorded in patients who undergo ventricular pacing from other sites. This could potentially lead to issues, such as ventricular under-sensing. Sensed R-wave amplitudes are significantly lower in the SCSP group at implant, and this difference can persist over long-term follow-up (**Table 2**). Many studies do not report these values at either implant or in the follow-up period, and this is something that should be emphasized and obligatorily reported in future publications.

Table 1
Patient demographics across current studies

Author, Year	Patient Number	Age, y (Mean ±SD)	Gender, Male (%)	Indication for Conduction System Pacing (His Bundle Pacing)
Deshmukh et al,[11] 2000	18	69 ± 10	—	AV node ablation • QRS <120 ms • Dilated cardiomyopathy • EF <40%
Moriña Vázquez et al,[45] 2001	12	—	—	AV node ablation • QRS <120 ms • Dilated cardiomyopathy • EF <40%
Zanon et al,[42] 2006	26	77 ± 5	19 (73)	AV nodal disease + sinus node dysfunction • Second-degree AVB (n = 11) • Paroxysmal third-degree AVB (n = 3) • Permanent AF with slow ventricular rate (n = 5) • SSS (n = 7)
Barba-Pichardo et al,[24] 2006	7	63–82 (range)	3 (43)	AV nodal disease • Syncope • Intraventricular conduction disturbance, • Infra-Hisian AV block • Left ventricular dyssynchrony
Catanzariti et al,[50] 2006	24	75.1 ± 6.4	13	AV nodal disease + sinus node dysfunction • SSS (n = 11) • AF with low EF (n = 7) • 2°–3° AV block (n = 5)
Occhetta et al,[51] 2007	68	79 ± 6	45(66)	AV node ablation (n = 52) • High ventricular rate, not controlled by pharmacologic therapy • Cardiomyopathy AV nodal disease (n = 16) • Sinus rhythm with 1°–2° or 3° AV block, all with narrow QRS complexes (<120 ms)
Zanon et al,[52] 2008	12	74 ± 9	9 (75)	AV nodal disease • AF with slow ventricular rate (n = 4) • Second-degree AV block (n = 6) • Third-degree AV block (n = 2)
Barba-Pichardo et al,[53] 2008	37	—	—	AV nodal disease • Supra-Hisian (n = 16) • Infra-Hisian (n = 21)
Lustgarten et al,[25] 2010	10	—	—	AV nodal disease/CRT (n = 10) • Cardiomyopathy • LBBB (n = 9), atypical RBBB (n = 1) • QRS >130 • NYHA class III
Barba-Pichardo et al,[44] 2010	91	74 ± 9.8	—	AV nodal
Kronborg et al,[54] 2011	38	67 ± 10	30 (79)	AV nodal disease • Second-degree AVB (n = 11) • Third-degree AVB (n = 16) • Second and third degree AVB (n = 11)
Barba-Pichardo et al,[55] 2013	16	67.56 ± 5.1	10 (62.5)	AV nodal disease/CRT (n = 16) • Cardiomyopathy • Dilated LV • NYHA class III

(continued on next page)

Table 1
(continued)

Author, Year	Patient Number	Age, y (Mean ±SD)	Gender, Male (%)	Indication for Conduction System Pacing (His Bundle Pacing)
Catanzariti et al,[56] 2012	26	71.6 ± 8.8	16 (61.5)	AV nodal disease + sinus node dysfunction • AF with slow ventricular rate (n = 7) • AVB block (n = 5) • SSS (n = 11)
Sharma et al,[57] 2015	94	74 ± 12	49 (65)	AV nodal disease • AVB block (n = 44) • SSS (n = 31)
Lustgarten et al,[58] 2015	29	71.33 (55.91–86.75)	19 (66)	AV nodal disease (n = 10) • Cardiomyopathy • LBBB (n = 28), atypical RBBB (n = 1) • QRS >130
Vijayaraman et al,[59] 2015	60	72 ± 15	33 (55%)	AV nodal disease + sinus node dysfunction • Sinus node dysfunction (n = 24) • AV conduction disease (n = 36)
Teng et al,[60] 2016	29	68 ± 13 y	16 (55)	AV nodal disease • LBBB (n = 29)
Su et al,[61] 2016	38	64.76 ± 10.85	25 (66)	AV nodal disease • AF with slow ventricular rate (n = 13) • QRS >130, with LBBB (n = 25)
Huang et al,[62] 2017	52	72.8 ± 8.3	26 (61.9)	AV node ablation for AF • NYHA II/III • HFpEF or HFrEF
Zhang et al,[63] 2017	39	S-HBP 64.5 ± 7.2 NS-HBP 64.3 ± 10.3	S-HBP 15 (65) NS-HBP 9 (64)	AV nodal disease + sinus node dysfunction • AF with slow ventricular rate (n = 28) • AVB (n = 3) • SSS (n = 6)
Shan et al,[64] 2017	16	70.6 ± 12.9	9 (56.3)	AV nodal disease + sinus node dysfunction • Sinus node dysfunction and/or AV conduction disease (n = 11) • QRS duration of ≥130 ms and LBBB with LVEF <35% (n = 4) • High-degree AVB with reduced EF (n = 1)
Ajijola et al,[65] 2017	21	62 ± 18	17 (80)	AV nodal disease/CRT • Bundle branch block with QRS >120 ms • NYHA class II–IV • EF <35%
Sharma et al,[29] 2017	106	71 ± 12	74 (70)	AV nodal disease • Cardiomyopathy with BBB (n = 48) • Cardiomyopathy with non-BBB (n = 17) • Paced rhythm and cardiomyopathy (n = 41)
Vijayaraman et al,[66] 2017	94	76 ± 11	58 (62)	AV nodal disease + sinus node dysfunction • AVB (n = 56) • SSS (n = 38)
Vijayaraman et al,[67] 2017	42	74 ± 11	19 (45)	AV node ablation

Abbreviations: AF, Atrial Fibrillation; AVB, Atrioventricular block; AV, AV node; HFpEF, heart failure with preserved ejection fraction; HFrEF, heart failure with reduced ejection fraction; NYHA, New York Heart Association; RBBB, right bundle branch block; S, sick sinus syndrome; S-HBP, Selective His bundle pacing; NS-HBP, Nonselective His bundle pacing.

Table 2
Lead sensing data

Author, Year	Sensing (mV)		Sensing for S-His Bundle Pacing (mV)		Sensing for NS-His Bundle Pacing (mV)	
	Acute	Follow-up	Acute	Follow-up	Acute	Follow-up
Deshmukh et al,[11] 2000	1.7 ± 0.7	2.2 ± 0.8	—	—	—	—
Moriña Vázquez et al,[45] 2001	—	—	—	—	—	—
Zanon et al,[42] 2006	2.9 ± 0.7	2.5 ± 1.8	—	—	—	—
Barba-Pichardo et al,[24] 2006	—	—	—	—	—	—
Catanzariti, 2006	4.31 ± 2.77	4.17 ± 3.6	—	—	—	—
Occhetta, 2007	—	—	—	—	—	—
Zannon, 2008	—	—	—	—	—	—
Barba-Pichardo et al,[44] 2010	—	—	—	—	—	—
Lustgarten et al,[25] 2010	—	—	—	—	—	—
Barba-Pichardo et al,[44] 2010	6.6 ± 1.5	5.1 ± 1.6	—	—	—	—
Kronborg, 2011	—	—	4.7 ± 4.7	3.0 ± 1.7	6.4 ± 4	6.8 ± 3.5
Barba-Pichardo, 2013	—	—	—	—	—	—
Catanzariti, 2013	2.8 ± 1.3	2.4 ± 1.4	—	—	—	—
Sharma, 2015	1.35 ± 0.9	—	—	—	—	—
Lustgarten, 2015	1.3	2.5	—	—	—	—
Vijayaraman, 2015	4.1 ± 2.8 (+ve HB injury group) 5.4 ± 3.2 (-ve HB injury group)	—	—	—	—	—
Teng, 2016	—	—	—	—	—	—
Su, 2016	Configuration 1 5.99 ± 4.12 Configuration 2 3.13 ± 1.26 Configuration 3 3.31 ± 1.92	Configuration 1 5.01 ± 3.45 Configuration 2 — Configuration 3 2.35 ± 1.65	—	—	—	—
Huang, 2017	3.7	2.1	—	—	—	—
Zhang, 2017	—	—	2.6 ± 1.5	—	5.8 ± 4.5	—
Ajijola, 2017	—	—	—	—	—	—
Sharma et al,[29] 2017	4 ± 3.4	5.4 ± 4.9	—	—	—	—
Shan, 2017	4.4 ± 5.3	4.3 ± 5.0	—	—	—	—
Vijayaraman, 2017	6.8 ± 5.3	7.2 ± 5.2	—	—	—	—
Vijayaraman, 2017	6.0 ± 5.9	5.1 ± 4.1	—	—	—	—

Abbreviations: NS-His, Non selective his bundle pacing; +ve, Positive; S-His, Selective his bundle pacing; −ve, negative.

Table 3
Lead pacing thresholds

Author, Year	Threshold (ms)	Thresholds, Volts (Means and SD, Unless Stated)		Threshold for S-His Bundle Pacing		Threshold for NS-His Bundle Pacing	
		Acute	Follow-up	Acute	Follow-up	Acute	Follow-up
Deshmukh et al,[11] 2000	0.5	2.4 ± 1.0	3.9 ± 2.5	—	—	—	—
Moriña Vázquez et al,[45] 2001	0.5	1.24 ± 0.13	1.31 ± 0.20	—	—	—	—
Zanon et al,[42] 2006	0.5	2.3 ± 1.0	2.8 ± 1.4	—	—	—	—
Barba-Pichardo et al,[24] 2006	0.4	1.2–2.3 (range)	Increased in 3 patients to 4, 4.5, and 4.5	—	—	—	—
Catanzariti, 2006	0.5	1.61 ± 0.55	1.71 ± 0.92	—	—	—	—
Occhetta, 2007	0.5	0.6 ± 0.3 V	0.9 ± 0.7	3.8	—	0.6 ± 0.3	1.0 ± 0.8
Zannon, 2008	0.5	2.18 ± 0.8	—	2.18 ± 0.8	—	—	—
Barba-Pichardo et al,[44] 2008	1.0	1.5 ± 0.9	—	—	—	—	—
Lustgarten et al,[25] 2010	0.5	3.1 ± 1.1	—	—	—	—	—
Barba-Pichardo, 2010	1.0	1.5 ± 0.8	1.3 ± 0.9 V	—	—	—	—
Kronborg, 2011	—	—	—	2.3 ± 1	2.1 ± 1.6	1.7 ± 1.5	1.8 ± 1.3
Barba-Pichardo, 2013	—	3.1 ± 0.44	3.7 ± 0.54	—	—	—	—
Catanzariti, 2013	0.5	1.9 ± 0.6	1.8 ± 0.7	—	—	—	—
Sharma, 2015	0.5	1.35 ± 0.9	1.50 ± 0.8	—	—	—	—

Study		1.3	2.5				
Lustgarten, 2015	—						
Vijayaraman, 2015	0.5	1.16 ± 0.4 (+ve HB injury group); 1.75 ± 0.7 (−ve HB injury group)	1.31 ± 0.6 (+ve HB injury group); 1.98 ± 0.9 (−ve HB injury group)	—	—	—	—
Teng, 2016	—	—	—	—	—	—	—
Su, 2016	—	Configuration 1 1.99 ± 0.85; Configuration 2 3.03 ± 1.44; Configuration 3 2.68 ± 1.11	Configuration 1 1.39 ± 0.77; Configuration 2 —; Configuration 3 2.27 ± 1.33	—	—	—	—
Huang, 2017	—	1.5 ± 1.0	1.5 ± 1.0	—	—	—	—
Zhang, 2017	—	—	—	1.6 ± 0.7	1.3 ± 0.8	1.0 ± 0.4	0.8 ± 0.5
Ajijola, 2017	0.6	1.9 ± 1.2	1.4 ± 0.8	—	—	—	—
Sharma et al,[29] 2017	1.0	1.4 ± 0.9	1.72 ± 1.4	—	—	—	—
Shan, 2017	—	0.9 ± 0.5	1.3 ± 0.8	—	—	—	—
Vijayaraman, 2017	—	1.35 ± 0.9	1.62 ± 1.0	—	—	—	—
Vijayaraman, 2017	—	1.0 ± 0.8	1.6 ± 1.2	—	—	—	—

Conduction system thresholds

High thresholds have been a significant backbone issue with SCSP (**Table 3**) and are expected given the stimulation of the ventricle through a fibrous sheath. Like sensing data, there is inconsistency in the current data regarding reporting of pacing thresholds, with a wide variation on reported pulse widths (0.4–1.0 ms). The larger pulse width is often selected because it has the ultimate goal of conserving longevity of battery by enabling lower pulse voltage to be delivered. Overall, based on the current data published, the threshold is higher than what is expected for the RV lead, with these thresholds continuing to elevate in some patients over longer follow-up periods. A threshold increase of greater than 1 V is considered significant and warrants further investigation. An observation of the authors (from the limited data) is that CSP is associated with lower thresholds, which could be seen as a potential advantage over SCSP. The mechanism behind increased thresholds overtime is likely related to fibrosis and possible microdislodgement of the lead.

Lead complication

In the studies published to date, lead complications seem higher than that expected with conventional RV or biventricular pacing (**Table 4**). There is also a relatively high incidence of lead dislodgement. Furthermore, many patients undergo generator change earlier than expected, likely a consequence of the high threshold. There are no reported cases, however, of perforation.

Outcomes

Overall, the data for SCSP are convincing for it's potential as both an alternative for an RV lead placement and CRT (**Table 5**). There is a significant amount of data showing preservation and improvement in left ventricular ejection fraction (LVEF), reduction in brain natriuretic peptide (BNP) levels and hospitalizations, increase in functional class, and improvement in mitral valve disease. Only a few select studies have addressed the issue of mortality, and further data are required in this regard. Also, there is a lack of data on hard endpoints comparing SCSP with CSP.

Lead extraction

There are no reports on lead extraction to date, and there is potential for injury to the cardiac skeleton on removal. This data will be required and will be an essential part of the patient-physician discussion when implanting these devices.

Difficult with conduction system recording/pacing

In 20% to 30% of cases, it is often tricky to obtain CSP and then insertion of the lead. This is likely a result of both the complexity of the lead placement combined with limited current lead technology. The authors imagine that in the future, these percentages will decrease.

Potential for injury

Lead placement in the HB region can result in damage to the bundles or AV node (**Fig. 9**). Many studies comment on either transient or permeant bundle branch block as a consequence of the insertion of the HBP lead. This is something that implanters need to be aware of and discuss with patients.

What Is Still Needed to Know?

As discussed previously, the data supporting CSP is relatively robust and provide good impetus for further clinical studies. There are a few critical issues, however, that need to be addressed. First, from an anatomic point of view, the depth and variation of the HB relative to the endocardial surface is not clear. Because there is only 1 particular type of lead depth (1.8 mm), standard population variability likely cannot be accommodated and this may have an impact on outcomes and results. Further studies need to examine this, and different variations in lead depth need to be created, with a goal of improving lead thresholds and battery longevity. Additionally, there needs to be an improvement in lead stability, and further mechanisms need to be explored in this regard. The development of strategies to identify patients for CSP and improved techniques to identify the CS with a low and stable CSP threshold will be beneficial. Lastly, new batteries that withstand higher energy output will significantly improve longevity.

Future clinical trials

Previously, the observational and small randomized studies that demonstrate improvement in LVEF, functional measures, and quality of life with CSP are discussed. The merits and demerits of any technology, however, must be evaluated through blinded and randomized clinical trials, powered for detection of hard clinical endpoints, before widespread adoption by all practitioners. The contemporary medical community demands rigor and improvement in the methodology of interventional trials, and there are an increasing number of sham-controlled trials in the literature (eg, SYMPLICITY and ORBITA). With these factors in mind, the questions about HBP that need to be addressed in multicenter,

Table 4
Outcomes of his bundle pacing leads

Study, Year	Lead Complications During Follow up, n (%)	Complication
Deshmukh et al,[11] 2000	2 (16)	• 1, high threshold • 1, lead dislodgement after 2 mo of implantation
Moriña Vázquez et al,[45] 2001	Not reported	
Zanon et al,[42] 2006	6 (35)	• 6, change the pacing configuration of the 3830 lead from bipolar to unipolar owing to under-sensing
Barba-Pichardo et al,[24] 2006	3	• 3, higher thresholds • No lead dislodgement was observed
Catanzariti, 2006	1	• 3, ventricular under-sensing, 1 at implant and 2 during follow-up
Occhetta, 2007	1 (1.5)	• 1, pacing lead slightly moved 3 cm from its original para-Hisian position
Zannon, 2008	Not reported	
Barba-Pichardo, 2008	Not reported	
Lustgarten et al,[25] 2010	Not reported	
Barba-Pichardo et al,[44] 2010	3 (3)	• 2, dislodged • 1, loss of capture
Kronborg, 2011	0 (0)	
Barba-Pichardo, 2013	0 (0)	
Barba-Pichardo, 2013	Not reported	
Catanzariti, 2013	3 (11)	• 3, elective replacement indicator at 30, 33, and 38 mo after implantation. In these patients, a high pacing output had to be programmed on implantation to obtain His bundle capture.
Sharma, 2015	3 (4)	• 3, ventricular lead revision (loss of capture in 2 and high threshold (>5 V at 0.5 ms) in 1)
Lustgarten, 2015	Not reported	
Vijayaraman, 2015	2 (3)	• 1, lead dislodgement due to ratcheting and required lead replacement at 4 mo • 1, HBP threshold increased from 1.25 V at implant to 3.5 V at 0.5 ms at 2 mo.
Teng, 2016	Not reported	
Su, 2016	Not reported	
Huang, 2017	5 (9.6)	• No lead dislodgement • 5, patients had an increase in HBP thresholds by at least 1 V over baseline thresholds
Zhang, 2017	Not reported	
Ajijola, 2017	1 (6)	• No lead dislodgement • 1, one patient lost nonselective His capture 1 mo after implant with a para-Hisian response due to a threshold increase to 3.5 V, which was restored with increased programmed output of 5 mV
Sharma et al,[29] 2017	10 (10)	• 7, increased thresholds • 3, loss of BBB recruitment • 1, device infection
Shan, 2017	0 (0%)	
Vijayaraman, 2017	12 (16)	• 5, revision (2 had loss of capture within 2 wk after implant; and progressive increase in pacing threshold (.5 V at 0.5 ms) at 2-y follow-up in 1 • 7, pacemaker generator change was performed in 7 patients due to early battery depletion
Vijayaraman, 2017	Not reported	

Table 5
Patient outcomes in reported studies of His bundle pacing

Study, Year	Outcome
Deshmukh et al,[11] 2000	• Reduction of LVESD and LVEDD • Increase in fractional shortening • LVEF improved • Improved NYHA functional class
Moriña Vázquez et al,[45] 2001	• Stabile LVDD and LVSD • Stabile EF
Zanon et al,[42] 2006	• Not addressed
Barba-Pichardo et al,[24] 2006	• Stabile EF, with improvement in 1 patient
Catanzariti, 2006	• Improved interventricular and intraventricular dyssynchrony • Improved mitral regurgitation
Occhetta, 2007	• Improved NYHA functional class • Improved quality of life • Improved 6-min walk test • Improved mitral regurgitation
Zannon, 2008	• Improved myocardial perfusion (Tc99m-SestaMIBI) • Improved mitral regurgitation
Barba-Pichardo, 2008	• Not addressed
Lustgarten et al,[25] 2010	• DHBP narrowed the QRS significantly compared with native conduction and biventricular
Barba-Pichardo et al,[44] 2010	• LVEF improved
Kronborg, 2011	• Narrow QRS
Barba-Pichardo, 2013	• Improved NYHA functional class • Improved LVEF • Reduction of LVESD and LVEDD • Reduced LA diameter
Catanzariti, 2013	• Improved interventricularand intraventricular dyssynchrony • Improved mitral regurgitation • Improved LVEF
Sharma, 2015	• Reduced risk of heart failure hospitalization • No improvement in mortality
Lustgarten, 2015	• Improved quality of life • Improved NYHA functional class • Improved LVEF
Vijayaraman, 2015	• Not addressed
Teng, 2016	• Not addressed
Su, 2016	• Not addressed
Huang, 2017	• Improved mitral valve regurgitation • Decreased LVEDD • Improved LVEF • Decreased serum BNP • Improved NYHA functional class • Reduced HFH
Zhang, 2017	• Not addressed
Ajijola, 2017	• Improved LVEF • Improved NYHA functional class
Sharma et al,[29] 2017	• Improved LVEF • Improved NYHA functional class

(continued on next page)

Table 5
(continued)

Study, Year	Outcome
Shan, 2017	• Improved mitral valve regurgitation • Decreased LVEDd • Improved LVEF • Decreased serum BNP • Improved NYHA functional class
Vijayaraman, 2017	• Reduced risk of death or HFH
Vijayaraman, 2017	• Improved LVEF • Improved NYHA functional class

Abbreviations: DHBP, Direct his bundle pacing; HFH, Heart failure hospitalization; LA, Left atrium; LVEDD, left ventricular end-diastolic diameter; LVEF, Left ventricular ejection fraction; LVESD, left ventricular end-systolic diameter; NYHA, New York Heart Association; Tc99m-Sestamibi, Technetium TC 99M Sestamibi.

double-blind, crossover, and randomized trials are as follows:

1. Is CSP noninferior/superior and safe, compared with CRT, for patients with a class I/IIa/IIb indication for CRT implantation?
2. Is CSP noninferior/superior and safe, compared with medical therapy, for patients with heart failure and reduced ejection fraction (EF) without a currently approved CRT indication?
3. Is CSP noninferior/superior and safe, compared with single/dual-chamber pacemaker, for patients with class I/IIa/IIb indications for single/dual-chamber pacing?

4. Finally, in these trials, and in large observational cohorts, what are the long-term lead related outcomes, such as pacing thresholds, lead stability, and battery life, with HBP, compared with conventional strategies?

A search for "His bundle" on clinicaltrials.gov yields 5 ongoing studies that are summarized in **Table 6**. These studies add to current understanding of the role of CSP. Several of these are multicenter and randomized, with crossover study arms, and there is 1 double-blind study as well. There are limited trials under way, however, that address hard clinical events as primary endpoints. There is a critical need to fund, design, and

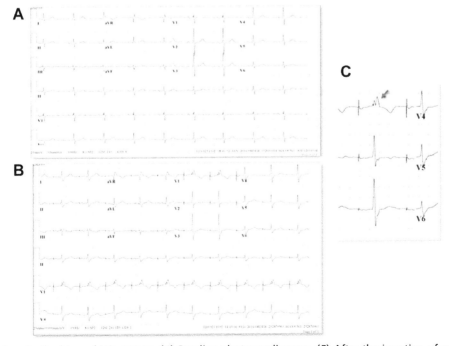

Fig. 9. Injury to the his purkinje system. (*A*) Baseline electrocardiogram. (*B*) After the insertion of an HB lead, there is development of an RBBB. (*C*) *Arrow* showing a close up of the new RBBB.

Table 6
Current his bundle pacing trials

Title	Design	Inclusion Criteria	Arms	Sponsor	Collaborators	Target Recruitment	Primary Outcome Measure	Estimated Study Completion
HOPE-HF (NCT02671903)	Multicenter, randomized, double-blind crossover	• EF<40% • NYHA II–IV • PR >200 • QRS <140 ms OR RBBB	AV optimized HBP vs backup pacing at 30 beats per minute	Imperial College London	• British Heart Foundation • Medtronic	160	Changes in exercise capacity using peak V_{O_2}	October 2019
Comparison of His Bundle Pacing and Bi-Ventricular Pacing in Heart Failure With Atrial Fibrillation (NCT02805465)	Multicenter, randomized, crossover	• Persistent AF undergoing AVNA • EF <40% • NYHA II–IV • QRS <120 ms	HBP vs CRT	First Affiliated Hospital of Wenzhou Medical University	• HT-Med Company • Chinese Academy of Medical Sciences, Fuwai Hospital • Shanghai Zhong-shan Hospital • Jiangsu People's Hospital • Wuhan Asia Heart Hospital • Sir Run Run Shaw Hospital • Shanxi People's Hospital	50	Change in EF	July 2018

His-SYNC (NCT02700425)	Multicenter, randomized, single blinded	Class I/IIa/IIb indication for CRT	HBP vs CRT	University of Chicago	• University of California, Los Angeles • Northwestern University • Rush University Medical Center	40	• Change in EF • Change in QRS duration • Time to first CV hospitalization or death	March 2021
His Bundle Pacing in Bradycardia and Heart Failure (NCT03008291)	Single center, observational	• EF <35% with CRT-P/D indication • AV block with dual chamber pacing indication	NA	Mayo Clinic	NA	40	QRS duration and morphology	December 2017
IMAGE-HBP (NCT03294317)	Observational	• Indication for single or dual chamber pacing (but not CRT)	NA	Medtronic Cardiac Rhythm and Heart Failure	NA	55	Implant success (H wave on EGM + threshold ≤2.5 V at 1 ms)	August 2019

conduct such studies, with close attention to trial design.

SUMMARY

CSP (HBP) is an intuitively attractive means for cardiac pacing. By using the native conduction system and thereby providing synchronous contraction, it has emerged as a pure physiologic form of pacing that has been shown safe and feasible in clinical practice. Benefits have been shown regarding improvement in LVEF, functional status, heart failure hospitalizations, and possibly mortality. Lead thresholds and lead stability represent leading barriers to current application, and further clinical studies need to show an established benefit over the conventional RV or biventricular pacing.

REFERENCES

1. Nathan DA, Center S, Wu CY, et al. An implantable synchronous pacemaker for the long term correction of complete heart block. Am J Cardiol 1963; 11:362–7.
2. Hochleitner M, Hortnagl H, Ng CK, et al. Usefulness of physiologic dual-chamber pacing in drug-resistant idiopathic dilated cardiomyopathy. Am J Cardiol 1990;66:198–202.
3. Hochleitner M, Hortnagl H, Hortnagl H, et al. Long-term efficacy of physiologic dual-chamber pacing in the treatment of end-stage idiopathic dilated cardiomyopathy. Am J Cardiol 1992;70:1320–5.
4. Wilkoff BL, Cook JR, Epstein AE, et al. Dual-chamber pacing or ventricular backup pacing in patients with an implantable defibrillator: the Dual Chamber and VVI Implantable Defibrillator (DAVID) Trial. JAMA 2002;288:3115–23.
5. Sweeney MO, Hellkamp AS, Ellenbogen KA, et al. Adverse effect of ventricular pacing on heart failure and atrial fibrillation among patients with normal baseline QRS duration in a clinical trial of pacemaker therapy for sinus node dysfunction. Circulation 2003;107:2932–7.
6. Connolly SJ, Kerr CR, Gent M, et al. Effects of physiologic pacing versus ventricular pacing on the risk of stroke and death due to cardiovascular causes. Canadian Trial of Physiologic Pacing Investigators. N Engl J Med 2000;342:1385–91.
7. Barsheshet A, Moss AJ, McNitt S, et al. Long-term implications of cumulative right ventricular pacing among patients with an implantable cardioverter-defibrillator. Heart Rhythm 2011;8:212–8.
8. Sweeney MO, Bank AJ, Nsah E, et al. Minimizing ventricular pacing to reduce atrial fibrillation in sinus-node disease. N Engl J Med 2007;357: 1000–8.
9. Gong X, Su Y, Liang Y, et al. Is right ventricular outflow tract pacing superior to right ventricular apex pacing? A long-term follow-up study. Int J Clin Exp Med 2017;10:5189–95.
10. Gong X, Su Y, Pan W, et al. Is right ventricular outflow tract pacing superior to right ventricular apex pacing in patients with normal cardiac function? Clin Cardiol 2009;32:695–9.
11. Deshmukh P, Casavant DA, Romanyshyn M, et al. Permanent, direct His-bundle pacing: a novel approach to cardiac pacing in patients with normal His-Purkinje activation. Circulation 2000;101:869–77.
12. Mulpuru SK, Cha Y-M, Asirvatham SJ. Synchronous ventricular pacing with direct capture of the atrioventricular conduction system: functional anatomy, terminology, and challenges. Heart Rhythm 2016; 13:2237–46.
13. His W Jr. The story of the atrioventricular bundle with remarks concerning embryonic heart activity. J Hist Med Allied Sci 1949;4:319–33.
14. Alanis J, Gonzalez H, Lopez E. The electrical activity of the bundle of His. J Physiol 1958;142:127–40.
15. James TN, Sherf L. Fine structure of the His bundle. Circulation 1971;44:9–28.
16. Chessa M, Giamberti A. The right ventricle in adults with tetralogy of fallot. Verlag (IL): Springer; 2012.
17. Scherlag BJ, Lazzara R. Is there longitudinal dissociation in the undamanged his bundle? In vitro studies in the normal canine heart. J Electrocardiol 2000;33:83–6.
18. Zhou P, Yang D, Liu P, et al. A method to find HIS bundle signals from surface ECG. Systems and Control in Aerospace and Astronautics, 2006 ISSCAA 2006 1st International Symposium on. 2006:3: p. 1457.
19. Chang Q, Liu R, Chen J. Surface electrocardiogram: could atrioventricular nodal and His bundle potentials be recorded beat by beat on "Saah electrocardiogram". Anatol J Cardiol 2017;18:110–4.
20. Kaufmann E, Rothberger C. Beiträge zur entstehungsweise extrasystolischer allorhythmien. Zeitschrift für die gesamte experimentelle Medizin 1919; 7:199.
21. Narula OS. Longitudinal dissociation in the His bundle. Br Heart J 1972;56(6):996–1006.
22. El-Sherif N, Amay-Y-Leon F, Schonfield C, et al. Normalization of bundle branch block patterns by distal His bundle pacing. Clinical and experimental evidence of longitudinal dissociation in the pathologic his bundle. Circulation 1978;57:473–83.
23. Puech P, Grolleau R, Morena H, et al. Improvement and normalisation of the QRS complex by stimulation of the bundle of His in complete left branch block. Arch Mal Coeur Vaiss 1979;72:815–24 [in French].
24. Barba-Pichardo R, Morina-Vazquez P, Venegas-Gamero J, et al. Permanent His-bundle pacing in

patients with infra-Hisian atrioventricular block. Rev Esp Cardiol 2006;59:553–8 [in Spanish].

25. Lustgarten DL, Calame S, Crespo EM, et al. Electrical resynchronization induced by direct His-bundle pacing. Heart Rhythm 2010;7:15–21.

26. Dabrowski P, Kleinrok A, Kozluk E, et al. Physiologic resynchronization therapy: a case of his bundle pacing reversing physiologic conduction in a patient with CHF and LBBB during 2 years of observation. J Cardiovasc Electrophysiol 2011;22:813–7.

27. Sharma PS, Huizar J, Ellenbogen KA, et al. Recruitment of bundle branches with permanent His bundle pacing in a patient with advanced conduction system disease: what is the mechanism? Heart Rhythm 2016;13:623–5.

28. Sharma PS, Dandamudi G, Herweg B, et al. Permanent His-bundle pacing as an alternative to biventricular pacing for cardiac resynchronization therapy: a multicenter experience. Heart Rhythm 2018;15(3):413–20.

29. Sharma PS, Ellison K, Patel HN, et al. Overcoming left bundle branch block by permanent His bundle pacing: evidence of longitudinal dissociation in the His via recordings from a permanent pacing lead. HeartRhythm Case Rep 2017;3:499–502.

30. Scherlag BJ, El-Sherif N, Hope RR, et al. The significance of dissociation of conduction in the canine His bundle. Electrophysiological studies in vivo and in vitro. J Electrocardiol 1978;11:343–54.

31. Scherlag BJ, Lazzara R. Functional aspects of His bundle physiology and pathophysiology: clinical implications. J Electrocardiol 2017;50:151–5.

32. Lazzara R, Yeh BK, Samet P. Functional transverse interconnections within the His bundle and the bundle branches. Circ Res 1973;32(4):509–15.

33. Friedman DJ, Hjorth MA, Sun AY, et al. Intermittent capture of the left bundle with permanent his bundle pacing: mechanistic insights and implications for an emerging field. J Cardiovasc Electrophysiol 2016; 27(11):1344–8.

34. Wikswo JP, Roth BJ. Virtual electrode theory of pacing cardiac bioelectric therapy. Boston, MA: Springer; 2009. p. 283–330.

35. Sepulveda NG, Roth BJ, Wikswo JP Jr. Current injection into a two-dimensional anisotropic bidomain. Biophys J 1989;55:987–99.

36. Stuckey J, Hoffman B, Kottmeier P, et al. Electrode identification of the conduction system during open heart surgery. Surg Forum 1958;9:202–4.

37. Scherlag BJ, Kosowsky BD, Damato AN. A technique for ventricular pacing from the His bundle of the intact heart. J Appl Physiol 1967;22: 584–7.

38. Narula OS, Scherlag BJ, Samet P. Pervenous pacing of the specialized conducting system in man. His bundle and A-V nodal stimulation. Circulation 1970;41:77–87.

39. Karpawich PP, Gates J, Stokes KB. Septal his-purkinje ventricular pacing in canines: a new endocardial electrode approach. Pacing Clin Electrophysiol 1992;15:2011–5.

40. Amitani S, Miyahara K, Sohara H, et al. Experimental his-bundle pacing: histopathological and electrophysiological examination. Pacing Clin Electrophysiol 1999;22:562–6.

41. Deshmukh P, Anderson K, Sayre P. Direct His bundle pacing: novel approach to permanent pacing in patients with severe ventricular dysfunction and atrial fibrillation. PACE 1996;19:700.

42. Zanon F, Baracca E, Aggio S, et al. A feasible approach for direct his-bundle pacing using a new steerable catheter to facilitate precise lead placement. J Cardiovasc Electrophysiol 2006;17:29–33.

43. Moriña Vázquez P, Barba-Pichardo R, Venegas-Gamero J, et al. Cardiac resynchronization through selective His bundle pacing in a patient with the so-called InfraHis atrioventricular block. Pacing Clin Electrophysiol 2005;28:726–9.

44. Barba-Pichardo R, Morina-Vazquez P, Fernandez-Gomez JM, et al. Permanent His-bundle pacing: seeking physiological ventricular pacing. Europace 2010;12:527–33.

45. Moriña Vázquez P, Barba Pichardo R, Venegas Gamero J, et al. Permanent pacing of the bundle of His after radiofrequency atrioventricular node ablation in patients with suprahisian conduction disturbances. Rev Esp Cardiol 2001;54:1385–93 [in Spanish].

46. Williams DO, Scherlag BJ, Hope RR, et al. Selective versus non-selective His bundle pacing. Cardiovasc Res 1976;10:91–100.

47. Vijayaraman P, Dandamudi G, Zanon F, et al. Permanent his bundle pacing: recommendations from a Multicenter His Bundle Pacing Collaborative Working Group for standardization of definitions, implant measurements, and follow-up. Heart Rhythm 2018; 15(3):460–8.

48. Linde C, Cleland JGF, Gold MR, et al. The interaction of sex, height, and QRS duration on the effects of cardiac resynchronization therapy on morbidity and mortality: an individual-patient data meta-analysis. Eur J Heart Fail 2018;20(4):780–91.

49. Biton Y, Zareba W, Goldenberg I, et al. Sex differences in long-term outcomes with cardiac resynchronization therapy in mild heart failure patients with left bundle branch block. J Am Heart Assoc 2015; 4(7) [pii:e002013].

50. Catanzariti D, Maines M, Cemin C, et al. Permanent direct his bundle pacing does not induce ventricular dyssynchrony unlike conventional right ventricular apical pacing. J Interv Card Electrophysiol 2006; 16(2):81–92.

51. Occhetta E, Bortnik M, Marino P, et al. Permanent parahisian pacing. Indian Pacing Electrophysiol J 2007;7(2):110–25.

52. Zanon F, Bacchiega E, Rampin L, et al. Direct His bundle pacing preserves coronary perfusion compared with right ventricular apical pacing: a prospective, cross-over mid-term study. Europace 2008;10(5):580–7.

53. Barba-Pichardo R, Moriña-Vázquez P, Venegas-Gamero J, et al. The potential and reality of permanent his bundle pacing. Rev Esp Cardiol 2008; 61(10):1096–9.

54. Kronborg MB1, Mortensen PT, Gerdes JC, et al. His and para-His pacing in AV block: feasibility and electrocardiographic findings. J Interv Card Electrophysiol 2011;31(3):255–62.

55. Barba-Pichardo R, Manovel Sánchez A, Fernández-Gómez JM, et al. Ventricular resynchronization therapy by direct His-bundle pacing using an internal cardioverter defibrillator. Europace 2013;15(1):83–8.

56. Catanzariti D, Maines M, Manica A, et al. Permanent His-bundle pacing maintains long-term ventricular synchrony and left ventricular performance, unlike conventional right ventricular apical pacing. Europace 2012;15(4):546–53.

57. Sharma PS, Dandamudi G, Naperkowski A, et al. Permanent His-bundle pacing is feasible, safe, and superior to right ventricular pacing in routine clinical practice. Heart Rhythm 2015;12(2):305–12.

58. Lustgarten DL, Crespo EM, Arkhipova-Jenkins I. His-bundle pacing versus biventricular pacing in cardiac resynchronization therapy patients: a cross-over design comparison. Heart Rhythm 2015;12(7): 1548–57.

59. Vijayaraman P1, Dandamudi G, Worsnick S, et al. Acute His-bundle injury current during permanent His-bundle pacing predicts excellent pacing outcomes. Pacing Clin Electrophysiol 2015;38(5): 540–6.

60. Teng AE, Lustgarten DL, Vijayaraman P. Usefulness of His bundle pacing to achieve electrical resynchronization in patients with complete left bundle branch block and the relation between native QRS axis, duration, and normalization. Am J Cardiol 2016;118(4):527–34.

61. Su L, Xu L, Wu SJ, et al. Pacing and sensing optimization of permanent His-bundle pacing in cardiac resynchronization therapy/implantable cardioverter defibrillators patients: value of integrated bipolar configuration. Europace 2016;18(9):1399–405.

62. Huang W, Su L, Wu S, et al. Benefits of permanent His bundle pacing combined with atrioventricular node ablation in atrial fibrillation patients with heart failure with both preserved and reduced left ventricular ejection fraction. J Am Heart Assoc 2017;6(4): e005309.

63. Zhang J, Guo J, Hou X, et al. Comparison of the effects of selective and non-selective His bundle pacing on cardiac electrical and mechanical synchrony. Europace 2018;20(6):1010–7.

64. Shan P, Su L, Zhou X, et al. Beneficial effects of upgrading to His bundle pacing in chronically paced patients with left ventricular ejection fraction< 50%. Heart Rhythm 2018;15(3):405–12.

65. Ajijola OA, Upadhyay GA, Macias C, et al. Permanent His-bundle pacing for cardiac resynchronization therapy: initial feasibility study in lieu of left ventricular lead. Heart Rhythm 2017;14(9):1353–61.

66. Vijayaraman P, Naperkowski A, Subzposh FA, et al. Permanent His bundle pacing: long-term lead performance and clinical outcomes. Heart Rhythm 2018;15(5):696–702.

67. Vijayaraman P, Subzposh FA, Naperkowski A. Atrioventricular node ablation and His bundle pacing. Europace 2017;19(suppl_4):iv10–6.

An Electro-Anatomic Atlas of His Bundle Pacing
Combining Fluoroscopic Imaging and Recorded Electrograms

Parikshit S. Sharma, MD, MPH, FACC, FHRS*,
Richard Trohman, MD, MBA

KEYWORDS

- Permanent His bundle pacing (HBP) • Anatomy of His bundle (HB) • Electro-anatomic map
- RAO and LAO views

KEY POINTS

- Permanent His bundle pacing (PHBP) has gained popularity as a promising tool for patients who need ventricular pacing.
- Understanding the anatomy of the His bundle (HB) region and the variations in its anatomy is critical to successful PHBP.
- Use of fluoroscopic right anterior oblique/left anterior oblique views can be very helpful in achieving better contact during implant and help prevent long-term issues, such as increasing capture thresholds.
- Careful mapping of the HB region with the lead can help in identification of level of disease/delay and successful implantation at a site distal to the site of disease.

INTRODUCTION

Permanent His bundle pacing (PHBP) was first described by Deshmukh and colleagues[1] in 2000. Since its original description, this technique has gained significant popularity. Better tools have improved implant success rates, and an increasing body of data now attests to the clinical benefits of PHBP.[2] In this article, the authors review relevant His bundle (HB) anatomy and link PHBP implant characteristics to patient anatomy using fluoroscopic and electro-anatomic correlations.

ANATOMY OF THE HIS BUNDLE

Wilhelm His Jr, a Swiss anatomist and cardiologist, described the HB in 1893 as a muscle bundle uniting the auricular and ventricular septal walls.[3] The atrioventricular (AV) node (AVN) was initially characterized by Sunao Tawara[4] in 1906 as a compact spindle-shaped network of cells arranged in a "knoten" (node) connected to the HB. Tawara's[4] original monograph "Das Reizleitungssystem des Saugetierherzens" ("The Stimulus Conducting System of Mammalian Hearts")[4] provided an exquisite morphologic description of

Disclosures: Dr P.S. Sharma: honoraria: Medtronic; consultant: St. Jude Medical. Dr R. Trohman: advisor: Boston Scientific/Guidant; research grants: Boston Scientific, Medtronic Inc, St. Jude Medical, Vitatron, and WyethAyerst/Wyeth Pharmaceuticals; consultant: Biosense Webster and St. Jude Medical; honoraria: Boston Scientific/Guidant CRM, Medtronic Inc, Daiichi-Sankyo, and St. Jude Medical.
Division of Cardiology, Rush University Medical Center, 1717 West Congress Parkway, Suite 300 Kellogg, Chicago, IL 60612, USA
* Corresponding author. Division of Cardiology, Rush University Medical Center, 1717 West Congress Parkway, Suite 300 Kellogg, Chicago, IL 60612, USA.
E-mail address: psharma.doc@gmail.com

Card Electrophysiol Clin 10 (2018) 483–490
https://doi.org/10.1016/j.ccep.2018.05.009
1877-9182/18/© 2018 Elsevier Inc. All rights reserved.

the AVN, HB, and surrounding atrial myocardium of 9 mammalian species, including humans.

The HB (named after Wilhelm His Jr) is now better characterized as a chordlike structure that traverses from the compact AVN through to the crest of the interventricular septum. The bundle of His, which measures an average of 1.8 cm in length with a width of 2 to 3 mm[5] and is composed of 2 distinct sections; the nonbranching (or penetrating) portion, which penetrates the fibrous AV ring and continues as the right bundle branch (RBB); and the branching portion of the His bundle from, which the branches of the left bundle originate[6] (Fig. 1).

The penetrating portion is about 5 to 10 mm in length and is related to the atrial part of the membranous septum (pars membranacea), the central fibrous body, the mitral ring, and the septal leaflet of the tricuspid valve. It pierces the collagenous central fibrous body of the heart and emerges at the level of the noncoronary aortic cusp below the posteroinferior edge of the membranous septum at its atrial portion before reaching the insertion of the septal leaflet of the tricuspid valve.[6]

The branching portion extends from the point where the bundle begins giving the most posterior fibers (actually the first fibers) of the left bundle branch (LBB) to the point that marks both, the most anterior strands of the LBB (the last ones), and the very beginning of the RBB. The branching segment runs on the crest of the interventricular septum lying on its left side with a variable length of about 5 to 10 mm leaving slender strands oriented inferiorly and slightly anteriorly on the left septal surface to form the LBB, whereas the RBB appears as a direct continuation of the HB[6] (see Fig. 1)

Anatomic Variations in His Bundle: Types of His Bundle

Kawashima and Sasaki[7] studied the macroscopic anatomy of the HB in 105 autopsied elderly human hearts. They described variability in the course of the HB relative to the membranous interventricular septum and noted 3 different anatomic variations (Fig. 2): (1) The most common (47% of the specimens) anatomic pattern (type I) was where the AV bundle ran along the lower border of the membranous septum and was usually covered with a thin layer of myocardial fibers; (2) type II was where the AV bundle was discretely separated from the membranous septum and insulated by thick myocardial fibers (32% of the specimens); and (3) type III (21% of the specimens) was where the AV bundle was naked and ran beneath the endocardium with no insulation from the surrounding myocardial fibers.[7] This variation is important to understand, as it is an important factor in achieving selective or nonselective PHBP.

Longitudinal Dissociation of the His Bundle

The concept of longitudinal dissociation within the HB was elegantly demonstrated by Narula[8] in

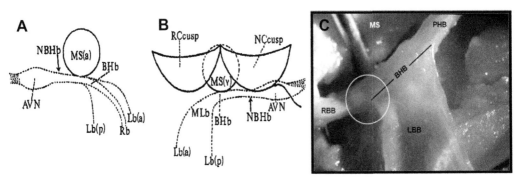

Fig. 1. Anatomy of the HB. (A) The structure of the AV node and HB as dissected from the right side of the AV septum. (B) The structure of the AV node and HB as dissected from the left side of the AV septum. (C) Preparation with amplification under stereoscopic dissecting microscope of the penetrating portion of the HB (PHB) and the left bundle branch (LBB) arising from the branching HB portion (BHB). The RBB appears as a continuation of the HB after the LBB has been given off. The circle points out the pseudobifurcation. The membranous septum (MS) has been separated from the summit of the ventricular septum. BHb, branching HB; Lb(a), origin of the anterior branches of the left bundle; Lb(p), origin of the posterior branches of the left bundle; MLb, main left bundle at its origin; MS(a), atrial MS; MS(v), ventricular MS; NBHb, nonbranching HB; NCcusp, noncoronary cusp of the aortic valve; Rb, right bundle (continuous extension of the HB); RCcusp, right coronary cusp (aortic valve). (*Adapted from* [A, B] Scherlag BJ, Lazzara R. Functional aspects of His bundle physiology and pathophysiology: clinical implications. J Electrocardiol 2017;50:151–5, with permission; and [C] Elizari MV. The normal variants in the left bundle branch system. J Electrocardiol 2017;50:389–99, with permission.)

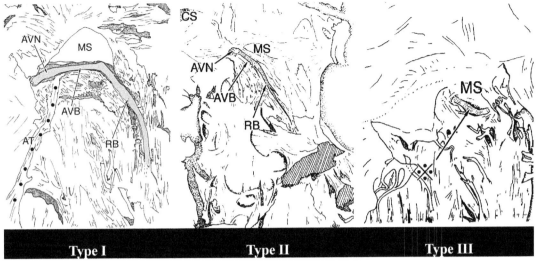

Fig. 2. Types of HB. Type I: The AV bundle runs along the lower border of the membranous septum (MS) and is covered with a thin layer of myocardial fibers. Type II: The AV bundle is discretely separated from the MS and insulated by thick myocardial fibers. Type III: The AV bundle is naked and runs beneath the endocardium with no insulation from the surrounding myocardial fibers. AVB, AV Bundle; CS, coronary sinus; RB, right bundle. (*Adapted from* Kawashima T, Sasaki H. A macroscopic anatomic investigation of atrioventricular bundle locational variation relative to the membranous part of the ventricular septum in elderly human hearts. Surg Radiol Anat 2005;27:206–13; with permission.)

1977. They postulated that delay or block within HB fibers could result in bundle branch block (BBB) and demonstrated that pacing distal to the site of conduction delay could recruit fibers predestined to be the bundle branches and, thereby, narrow the QRS duration. El-Sherif[9] demonstrated similar findings in an experimental model. Understanding that BBB or delay can be within predestined HB fibers and that pacing distal to the site of disease/delay might overcome BBB patterns and narrow the QRS formed the basis for PHBP (**Fig. 3**). The authors highlight this concept in some of their reports[10,11] and a recent multicenter experience of 106 patients.[12] Case 3 discussed later also demonstrates this physiology.

PERMANENT HIS BUNDLE PACING

PHBP was first described in clinical practice in 2000 by Deshmukh and colleagues.[1] PHBP was successful in 12 of 18 patients (67%) with chronic atrial fibrillation (AF), left ventricular ejection fraction less than 40%, and a QRS duration less than 120 milliseconds after ablation of the AV junction. Over the past 2 decades, with improvement in implant tools, PHBP has been performed with a higher success rate (80%–90%) and data have emerged on improved clinical outcomes in comparison with conventional right ventricular (RV) apical pacing.[2,12–16] More recent data suggest the feasibility of PHBP for cardiac resynchronization therapy (CRT) either as a rescue strategy

when a coronary sinus lead implantation fails or as a primary CRT strategy.

Permanent His Bundle Pacing and Its Relationship to the Tricuspid Valve

The location of the implanted HBP lead and its relationship to the tricuspid annulus (TA) have been described in a few reports. In a postmortem study of an elderly woman with a previously implanted HBP lead, Correa de Sa and colleagues[17] demonstrated that the lead tip was unequivocally implanted on the atrial side of the TA. Vijayaraman and colleagues[18] performed an imaging evaluation of a middle-aged man with an HBP lead and similarly demonstrated that the lead tip was on the atrial aspect of the tricuspid valve plane. As noted earlier, given that most of the penetrating HB is on the atrial aspect of the septal leaflet of the tricuspid valve, if conduction system disease is more proximal within the AVN or the penetrating portion of the HB, the lead tip could possibly be located on the atrial aspect of the TA. Whether this is always the case, particularly in cases whereby the disease is more distal, remains unanswered. Logically, the appropriate lead tip location would likely depend on the level of disease within the HB.

MAPPING THE HIS BUNDLE

Traditionally, mapping of the HB has been performed using multipolar mapping catheters

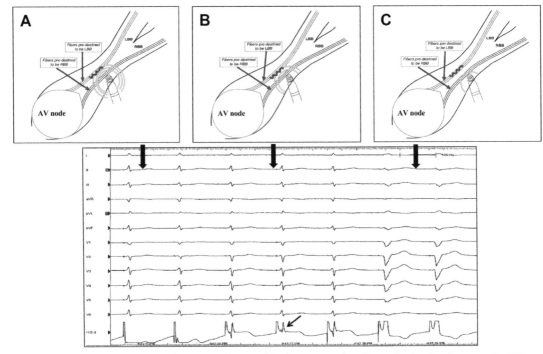

Fig. 3. Longitudinal dissociation of the HB. Fibers within the HB are already predestined to become the RBB and LBB as depicted. If there is localized disease within the fibers predestined to be the LBB (demonstrated in image), placing the lead at or distal to the site of delay/disease might overcome left BBB (LBBB). (*A*) Pacing at 2.0 V results in capture of local ventricular tissue and His (both RBB and LBB fibers). (*B*) Pacing at 1.5 V results in selective His capture (both RBB and LBB fibers) with loss of ventricular capture (*arrow* shows discrete local electrogram in the HBP lead). (*C*) Pacing at 1.0 V demonstrates capture of RBB fibers alone with LBBB pattern. (*Adapted from* Sharma PS, Dandamudi G, Herweg B, et al. Permanent His-bundle pacing as an alternative to biventricular pacing for cardiac resynchronization therapy: a multicenter experience. Heart Rhythm 2018;15(3):413–20; with permission.)

(inferior approach via femoral venous or superior approach via axillary/internal jugular vein). This method would help one identify the level of block: AVN, intra-Hisian (likely underestimated), and infra-Hisian. However, with the available tools for PHBP, using a preformed delivery sheath (C315, Medtronic, Minneapolis, MN) and a lead (3830, Medtronic, Minneapolis, MN), mapping of the HB region can usually be performed by recording unipolar electrograms from the lead tip. The intracardiac recordings can be displayed either on the Electrophysiology mapping system by using alligator cables or directly on a pacing system analyzer with a sweep speed of 50 mm/s. A mapping catheter can be used in cases whereby it is challenging to find the HB using the PHBP delivery system and lead.

Using Fluoroscopic Views During Permanent His Bundle Pacing

Traditionally, mapping of the HB is performed in the right anterior oblique (RAO) view. This view allows an anterior and posterior orientation with the RV and right atrium (RA) and helps localize the TA plane. Pulling back the system (lead and sheath) from the RV to the RA helps localize the TA. Once one gets to the TA, fine motions allow HB potential localization.

The left anterior oblique (LAO) view is underutilized during PHBP. However, the LAO view can provide better insight into septal contact. If the system (sheath and lead tip) moves from superior and inferior, contact might be inadequate, whereas right to left movement with the septum suggests better contact (**Fig. 4**).

Fluoroscopic views are also important in assessing lead slack after lead fixation. In the RAO view, the HB lead should have a loop like an atrial lead (**Fig. 5**). Too much slack (if the lead is bouncing in and out of the RV) might be detrimental because this would cause stress on the lead and the lead tip with tricuspid valve motion. This stress could, over time, lead to microdislodgements and increased capture thresholds.

In patients with atrial dilation and cardiomyopathy, the HB can migrate more superiorly or inferiorly to the expected location. Using the

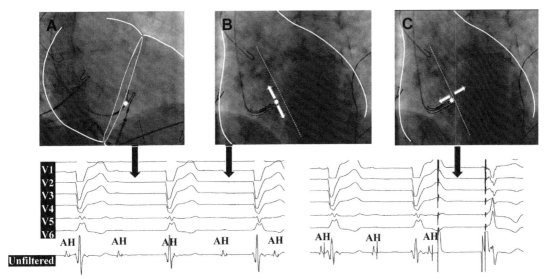

Fig. 4. Mapping the HB: Use of RAO/LAO views. (*A*) RAO view of the mapping system (fixed curve sheath and lead in a unipolar fashion) at the TA with corresponding electrograms. (*B*) LAO view of the same location with the same torque on the system. As depicted in the image, the system fails to make adequate contact with the septum. As a consequence, the lead tip moves superior and inferior, independent of septal motion (*upward and downward arrows*). The corresponding HB electrogram is small in amplitude with suggestion of HV block. (*C*) LAO view with more counterclockwise torque on the system and the lead extended out of the sheath demonstrating better contact with the septum. This view results in a larger HB electrogram recording as noted and motion of the system from left to right in synchrony with the septum (*rightward and leftward arrows*). Pacing at this site narrows the QRS and overcomes the baseline left BBB (LBBB).

deflectable (C304, Medtronic Inc, Minneapolis, MN) sheath might help better localize the HB and lead to a successful implant if the standard fixed-curve sheath fails to find the HB.

Prosthetic valves might also act as a marker to help localize the HB. The authors published their experience with PHBP in patients with various prosthetic valves and demonstrated a success rate of 93% (28 of 30 patients).[19] The prosthetic valves act as fluoroscopic markers to help localize the HB location with an average distance of 14 mm inferior to an aortic valve replacement (AVR) and 19 mm distal to a tricuspid valve ring. The only patients one should be careful with PHBP are

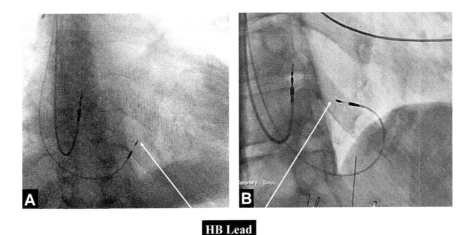

Fig. 5. Importance of lead slack. A 64-year-old gentleman with advanced AV block underwent a dual-chamber PHBP and developed progressive increase in HB capture threshold from 1 V at 1 millisecond to 3.5 V at 1 millisecond over a 10-month period. (*A*) Baseline lead slack after initial implant. (*B*) HB lead slack pulled into the RV at time of HB lead revision. On adjusting the lead slack, HB capture threshold improved instantly to 2.5 V at 1 millisecond and continued to improve to 1.5 V at 1 millisecond on postrevision day 1.

patients with a CoreValve (Medtronic, Minneapolis, MN) transcatheter AVR (TAVR). The risk of AV block is greater with the CoreValve, attributed to valve design and the potential deeper implantation into the left ventricular outflow tract. This deeper implantation may result in increased injury to the distal HB and LBBs, which may be delayed because of the self-expanding nature of the prosthesis and tissue edema. This delay could, theoretically, result in an inability to recruit the HB.[19]

CASE EXAMPLES

Case 1: Permanent His Bundle Pacing in Intra-Hisian Disease with Narrow QRS

A 76-year-old man with a known history of hypertension presented with symptomatic 2:1 AV block and a narrow QRS (98 milliseconds). He underwent an attempt at a dual-chamber pacemaker with PHBP. Proximal HB mapping revealed an

HV of 82 milliseconds (**Fig. 6**A) on the conducted beats, whereas distal HB mapping revealed AH block with an HV interval of 44 milliseconds (**Fig. 6**B) suggestive of intra-Hisian delay of 38 milliseconds. The lead implanted at the distal HB (**Fig. 6**C) resulted in selective HBP morphology.

Case 2: Permanent His Bundle Pacing in Patient with Edwards Sapien Transcatheter Aortic Valve Replacement

An 85-year-old woman with a known history of hypertension and aortic stenosis with right BBB (RBBB) at baseline (QRSd 140 milliseconds, **Fig. 7**A) undergoes an (Edwards Lifesciences Corp., Irvine, CA) TAVR valve. After the procedure, she developed complete heart block and needed a temporary screw-in pacemaker (paced QRSd 180 milliseconds, **Fig. 7**B). Given persistent AV block without recovery, she underwent a dual-

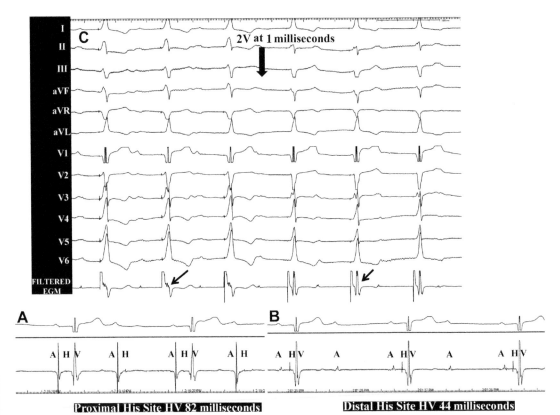

Fig. 6. PHBP in a patient with intra-Hisian disease. (*A*) Electrograms obtained from the HBP lead during mapping in the proximal HB region demonstrated 2:1 HV block and HV interval of 82 milliseconds. (*B*) At a slightly distal location (5 mm), 2:1 AH block (no His deflection following non-conducted atrial electrogram) is noted with a shorter HV interval of 44 milliseconds confirming that the level of block is intra-Hisian. (*C*) Transition from non-selective to selective His capture with decreasing output at 2 V at 1 millisecond (Arrows represent local septal ventricular capture suggesting non-selective capture followed by loss of ventricular capture with selective capture at outputs below 2V @ 1ms). (*Adapted from* Sharma PS, Dandamudi G, Herweg B, et al. Permanent His-bundle pacing as an alternative to biventricular pacing for cardiac resynchronization therapy: a multicenter experience. Heart Rhythm 2018;15(3):413–20; with permission.)

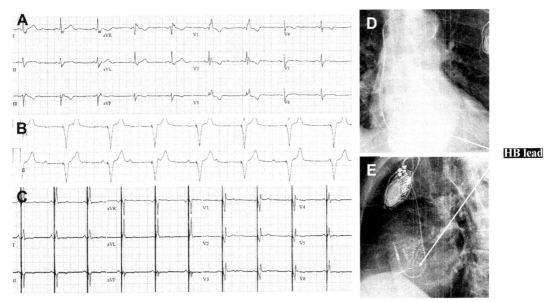

Fig. 7. PHBP in a patient with TAVR. (*A*) Baseline electrocardiogram with QRSd of 140 milliseconds. (*B*) After TAVR with RV apical pacing (180 milliseconds). (*C*) After PHBP with QRSd of 88 milliseconds. (*D, E*) Fluoroscopic views in posteroanterior and left lateral projections demonstrating the tip of the HB lead (*arrows*) located distal to the Edwards Sapien TAVR valve. CHB, complete heart block.

chamber pacemaker implant with PHBP, which overcame RBBB (HBP QRSd 88 milliseconds, **Fig. 7**C). Fluoroscopic images demonstrated the site of successful PHBP distal to the edge of the ES TAVR valve (**Fig. 7**D, E).

Case 3: Permanent His Bundle Pacing in Intra-Hisian Disease with Left Bundle Branch Block

A 79-year-old man with a history of hypertension and type II diabetes was admitted with dizziness

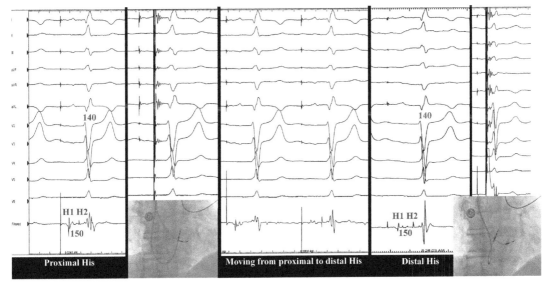

Fig. 8. PHBP in a patient with intra-Hisian block and LBBB. Proximal HB electrograms demonstrate a split HB (H1-H2 of 150 milliseconds). RAO fluoroscopic view demonstrates location of the tip electrode. Pacing at this site demonstrates a similar QRS with LBB delay. Moving from proximal to distal HB position results in a distal site that in 0.5 cm more distal fluoroscopically with a larger distal HB electrogram. Pacing at this site results in narrowing of the QRS and loss of LBB delay. Please note there is no local ventricular capture suggesting selective HB capture and LBB recruitment. (*Adapted from* Sharma PS, Ellison K, Patel HN, et al. Overcoming left bundle branch block by permanent His bundle pacing: evidence of longitudinal dissociation in the His via recordings from a permanent pacing lead. HeartRhythm Case Rep 2017;3:499–502; with permission.)

and fatigue in the setting of sinus node dysfunction with junctional rhythm in the 30s. He was also noted to have a rate-related delay in the LBB at 60 bpm. Given the left BBB (LBBB), the authors planned for an HBP lead implant with an attempt to recruit the LBB delay.

The authors started with implantation of the atrial lead in order to unmask the rate-related delay in LBB. **Fig. 8** demonstrates HB recordings and pace mapping (5 V at 1 millisecond) at different HB sites. The final location of the HB lead resulted in selective HBP with recruitment of the LBBB and narrowing of the QRS to 90 milliseconds.

SUMMARY

PHBP has emerged as a promising technique for patients who need ventricular pacing. Understanding the anatomy of the HB region and the variations in the anatomy of this region is key not only to achieve successful PHBP but also to define the type of PHBP achieved (selective or nonselective). Careful mapping of the HB region with the lead can help in identification of the level of disease/delay and result in successful implantation at a site distal to the site of disease.

ACKNOWLEDGMENTS

The authors thank Dr Pugazhendhi Vijayaraman and Dr Kenneth Ellenbogen for their continued mentorship.

REFERENCES

1. Deshmukh P, Casavant DA, Romanyshyn M, et al. Permanent, direct his-bundle pacing: a novel approach to cardiac pacing in patients with normal his-purkinje activation. Circulation 2000;101:869–77.
2. Sharma PS, Ellenbogen KA, Trohman RG. Permanent his bundle pacing: the past, present, and future. J Cardiovasc Electrophysiol 2017;28:458–65.
3. WH Jr. The function of the embryonic heart and its significance in the interpretation of the heart action in the adult (translated from German). Arbeiten Aus der Med Klin zu Leipzig 1983;1983(1):14–50.
4. Tawara S. Das Reizleitungssystem des Saugetierherzens. Eine anatomisch-histologische Studie fiber das Atrioventrikularbiindel und die Purkinjeschen Faden. Jena (Germany): Gustav Fischer; 1906. p. 135–8.
5. Scherlag BJ, Lazzara R. Functional aspects of His bundle physiology and pathophysiology: clinical implications. J Electrocardiol 2017;50:151–5.
6. Elizari MV. The normal variants in the left bundle branch system. J Electrocardiol 2017;50:389–99.
7. Kawashima T, Sasaki H. A macroscopic anatomical investigation of atrioventricular bundle locational variation relative to the membranous part of the ventricular septum in elderly human hearts. Surg Radiol Anat 2005;27:206–13.
8. Narula OS. Longitudinal dissociation in the His bundle. Bundle branch block due to asynchronous conduction within the His bundle in man. Circulation 1977;6:996–1006.
9. El-Sherif N. Normalization of bundle branch block patterns by distal his bundle pacing. clinical and experimental evidence of longitudinal dissociation in the pathologic his bundle. Circulation 1978;57: 473–83.
10. Sharma PS, Huizar J, Ellenbogen KA, et al. Recruitment of bundle branches with permanent His bundle pacing in a patient with advanced conduction system disease: what is the mechanism? Heart Rhythm 2016;13:623–5.
11. Sharma PS, Ellison K, Patel HN, et al. Overcoming left bundle branch block by permanent His bundle pacing: evidence of longitudinal dissociation in the His via recordings from a permanent pacing lead. HeartRhythm Case Rep 2017;3:499–502.
12. Sharma PS, Dandamudi G, Herweg B, et al. Permanent His-bundle pacing as an alternative to biventricular pacing for cardiac resynchronization therapy: a multicenter experience. Heart Rhythm 2018;15(3):413–20.
13. Sharma PS, Dandamudi G, Naperkowski A, et al. Permanent His-bundle pacing is feasible, safe, and superior to right ventricular pacing in routine clinical practice. Heart Rhythm 2015;12:305–12.
14. Lustgarten DL, Crespo EM, Arkhipova-Jenkins I, et al. His-bundle pacing versus biventricular pacing in cardiac resynchronization therapy patients: a crossover design comparison. Heart Rhythm 2015; 12:1548–57.
15. Vijayaraman P, Dandamudi G, Zanon F, et al. Permanent his bundle pacing: recommendations from a multicenter his bundle pacing collaborative working group for standardization of definitions, implant measurements, and follow-up. Heart Rhythm 2018; 15(3):460–8.
16. Ajijola OA, Upadhyay GA, Macias C, et al. Permanent His-bundle pacing for cardiac resynchronization therapy: initial feasibility study in lieu of left ventricular lead. Heart Rhythm 2017;14(9):1353–61.
17. Correa de Sa DD, Hardin NJ, Crespo EM, et al. Autopsy analysis of the implantation site of a permanent selective direct his bundle pacing lead. Circ Arrhythm Electrophysiol 2012;5:244–6.
18. Vijayaraman P, Dandamudi G, Bauch T, et al. Imaging evaluation of implantation site of permanent direct His bundle pacing lead. Heart Rhythm 2014; 11:529–30.
19. Sharma PS, Subzposh FA, Ellenbogen KA, et al. Permanent His-bundle pacing in patients with prosthetic cardiac valves. Heart Rhythm 2017;14:59–64.

His Bundle Pacing
Getting on the Learning Curve

Daniel L. Lustgarten, MD, PhD, FHRS

KEYWORDS

- His bundle pacing • Training • Expertise • Competence • Physiologic pacing

KEY POINTS

- His bundle pacing procedure requires higher level of expertise compared with standard pacing techniques.
- It is important for the implanter to have a solid understanding of electrophysiological (EP) mapping.
- Given our current level of understanding regarding electrical dyssynchrony, it is important for implanters to have expertise in all forms of cardiac pacing.
- Mastering His bundle pacing can be readily achieved with good foundations in implant techniques and EP anatomy and mapping.

INTRODUCTION

In order to provide perspective on the skill sets required to become facile with His bundle pacing (HBP), it is useful to consider it more broadly in the context of cardiac pacing, which developed from a surgical procedure to an invasive vascular one, with the skill sets transitioning from the surgical operating room to the cardiac catheterization and electrophysiology (EP) laboratories.[1–3] Minor surgical skills had to be developed early in this transition by cardiologists and subsequently electrophysiologists advantaged relative to the surgeon with a working knowledge of relational fluoroscopic anatomy and the disease processes being treated by pacemakers. Coupling those procedural skills with a more focused understanding of subsequent clinical management of chronically implanted devices placed implantable cardiac devices even more squarely in the realms of cardiology and EP. In this context, HBP can be thought of as the next step in the evolving field of cardiac pacing, requiring all of the prior skill sets but adding to that a thorough understanding of the EP anatomy of the atrioventricular (AV) junction and the patterns of activation that are consequent to

implantation of a permanent pacing lead into the AV junction. A deep knowledge of EP anatomy and His Purkinje disease is necessary to perform this procedure well and to maximize the probability of excellent long-term care of the patient. In this article, the author delineates some of the critical aspects of HBP that differentiate it from its device therapy antecedents, thereby providing the reader a sense of what tools they will need to develop or acquire in order to do this procedure well. We will first consider technical aspects and then look at the EP foundational knowledge that should be developed by the operator. Finally, the author provides a perspective on the numbers of procedures that may be required to become competent as a His bundle system implanter.

TECHNICAL CONSIDERATIONS

HBP is distinguished from standard pacing by the need for an electrogram acquisition system that permits identification of the His potential, which in most instances will be evident on the pacing electrode when sensing a conducted or junctional escape beat. One must therefore have familiarity with real-time observation and interpretation of

The University of Vermont School of Medicine, The University of Vermont Medical Center, 111 Colchester Avenue, McClure 1 Cardiology, Burlington, VT 05401, USA
E-mail address: daniel.lustgarten@uvmhealth.org

Card Electrophysiol Clin 10 (2018) 491–494
https://doi.org/10.1016/j.ccep.2018.05.012

intracardiac electrograms. Although it is possible to use a standard pacing system analyzer, a multichannel system allows attachment of 12 lead surface electrodes and provides better electrogram resolution and more flexible options for sweep speeds and filtering. In addition, a multichannel mapping system allows for the addition of a multipolar His mapping EP catheter, which can be very helpful, especially for one who is just learning the technique, to map the His along most of its length and provide a fluoroscopically obvious demonstration as to where the His lead delivery sheath needs to be manipulated in order to secure it at or very near the His bundle.[4] As one becomes more familiar with the behavior of the delivery sheath, the need for an EP catheter becomes less critical, although it can be helpful in cases where for one reason or another mapping the His is challenging. In addition, a multichannel system permits 12-lead surface electrocardiogram acquisition: the 12 lead helps define clearly the pacing response for different outputs and/or polarities at any given site along the length of the His bundle. This is particularly important when mapping and pacing into diseased His Purkinje tissue, wherein subtle morphology shifts can be readily detected and may be meaningful in terms of anticipated clinical response. As will be discussed later, this latter point is one of the most substantive distinguishing characteristics of HBP relative to right ventricle pacing, where QRS morphology is not a consideration, or left ventricle (LV) lead placement, which is constrained by available anatomic targets.

Pacing lead delivery options are currently limited and described in detail in Faiz A. Subzposh and Pugazhendhi Vijayaraman's article, "Long-Term Results of His Bundle Pacing," in this issue. Although lead delivery can be performed by hand shaping stylets, lead delivery sheaths allow greater control and precision and mastering their use is central to performing this procedure successfully. Although experience with slit-able LV lead delivery sheaths is helpful, the purpose of the sheath is subtly but importantly different. In the case of LV leads the sheaths serve as support, whereas the His bundle sheaths provide control for precise targeting and mapping. There are specific hand motions that determine motion and positioning: understanding and internalizing these motions represent the critical technical aspects of the procedure that conscribe most of the HBP learning curve. Specifically, with the 6-Fr stiff preshaped C315 His sheath very small motions can cause dramatic position changes, with clockwise rotation sending the system anteriorly and toward the ventricle, with counterclockwise rotation rotating the sheath posteriorly and toward the

atrium. These motions provide critical feedback to the operator regarding the reach required to adequately map along the length of the AV junction from its atrio-posterior extent (closer to the AV node) to its most anterior-ventricular aspect adjacent or within the membranous septum. Difficulties encountered may be addressed either by hand shaping the sheath for more anterior reach or by choosing to switch to a deflectable sheath. The advantage of the deflectable sheath is that it can help provide more anterior reach and the curve can be modified to target more distally or proximally. The disadvantage is the absence of a septal plane of deflection, making it more difficult at times to get the lead screw to catch: often a fair amount of counterclockwise torque is needed to try to catch the endocardium. At times, however, the tip of the sheath will seat well at the nexus between Todaro tendon and the tricuspid valve (TV) annulus, where often an excellent His pacing response and threshold can be obtained. Typically, if there is no further advantage noted using this sheath within 10 to 15 minutes it is reasonable to consider an alternative pacing strategy. If the issue is finding a His potential, before giving up it can sometimes be helpful to place an octapolar His mapping catheter from an adjacent axillary sheath and use that to target electrode bipoles recording a distinct His potential.

Contending with HBP thresholds represents another novel aspect of the procedure in that pacing thresholds tend to be higher relative to standard pacing sites, and there can be uniquely rapid and dramatic changes in thresholds—usually for the better, but not always—at a given pacing site. There are at least 2 factors to take into account that need to be understood: one is learning to record and recognize His injury current, the presence of which is reassuring for long-term stable capture.[5] The second is to be aware of how the lead moves at the implant site; although not proved yet in this author's personal experience, significant motion of the lead tip likely indicates the implant site is very close to or potentially through the base of the septal TV leaflet and is at higher risk for microdislodgement. Others have observed that wide differences in capture threshold between unipolar and bipolar vectors may also predict future threshold increases and probably warrants repositioning.

ELECTROPHYSIOLOGICAL FOUNDATIONAL KNOWLEDGE

The fact that there is a specific EP target distinguishes HBP from any other form of permanent pacing, and as such is the aspect that may pose the greatest challenge for implanters new to the technique. The process involved in a successful implantation requires mapping the His potential and developing an intimate understanding of the various pacing patterns encountered and the relational anatomy of a given site. Mapping in the context of a His bundle implant is different from EP studies in that (a) mapping is being performed from above through an open incision, whereas typically in EP studies and ablations mapping is done from the femoral approach; (b) access to an EGM acquisition system other than a PSA may be difficult in laboratories where implants are done separately from the ablation laboratory; (c) the process of mapping involves familiarity with a unique set of tools and connections, and currently is limited to basically two sheath designs, neither of them ideal; and (d) because the intention is to leave the lead permanently implanted, the objective of mapping is to find a site with adequate threshold and where oversensing of atrial electrograms will not result in inappropriate inhibition of the His lead.

Once the lead is actively fixed, there should be clear demonstration of the type of His bundle capture present with documentation of the relevant thresholds for each pattern encountered. The fact that multiple patterns of capture can be encountered is perhaps the most nuanced aspect of HBP—in truth there are patterns of activation that are still not completely understood—and having a working knowledge of these patterns is central to maximizing the potential benefits of HBP.[4]

When one is first learning HBP it makes sense to start with normal His Purkinje conduction patients, because deviations from a normal narrow QRS morphology are most readily apparent in these patients and there is a lower probability of causing intermittent heart block as one maps. As described in Faiz A. Subzposh and Pugazhendhi Vijayaraman's article, "Long-Term Results of His Bundle Pacing," in this issue, there are 2 basic paced morphologies encountered in patients with normal conduction, selective and nonselective capture. However, these 2 patterns are encountered in at least 2 different scenarios that are contingent on the underlying AV junctional anatomy, which varies between individuals, and the relative placement of the pacing lead. Sober reflection and mastery of these patterns and anatomic variation in the context of a paper or textbook are a good starting point, but the HBP lead implanter has to develop sufficient understanding of these patterns to recognize them on the fly and to be able to make important choices that will determine the procedure outcome. It is helpful to use a triggered review screen so that changes in capture morphology can be immediately appreciated, as can the relative size of local and/or far-field electrograms that can lead to inappropriate oversensing etc.

The presence of underlying conduction disease adds a significant layer of complexity to the procedure. As discussed elsewhere in this book, HBP can treat underlying complete or high-grade heart block with or without His Purkinje abnormalities and can in effect bypass the apparent level of block by reengaging previously latent His Purkinje tissue.[1,6] However, there are multiple issues that lend this patient population to a fair amount of nuanced interpretation. In spite of the original publication by Narula on longitudinal dissociation,[7] output-dependent fascicular capture has been clearly demonstrated in the context of active-fixation pacing leads[1]: maximal resynchronization threshold needs to be clearly defined at the time of implant and during all subsequent follow-up, which requires the operator to be able to distinguish the QRS morphologies observed during threshold testing.

Furthermore, if a given site does not elicit QRS normalization, it is possible in some cases, consistent with Narula's observations,[7] to find more distal sites wherein normalization of the QRS is possible. However, if the lead is very close or potentially even screwed through part of septal valve leaflet, there may be increased lead tip motion and this may increase the possibility of subsequent microdislodgement.

The number of cases it will take to become comfortable with the procedure is going to vary depending on an operator's training and experience: for operators who have spent a lot of time in the EP laboratory doing EP studies and ablations, who also have considerable implant experience, a handful of cases may be more than enough to feel comfortable with the procedure. Conversely if someone is coming to the procedure with asymmetry in their expertise, it is going to take more cases to gain the experience necessary to make the procedure start to feel more routine. Given limited tools currently available, some cases remain extremely difficult even after years of experience, and when encountering difficulties, the better part of valor often demands converting to a traditional implant and/or use of an LV lead. The total number of cases one should do to demonstrate and maintain competence ultimately can and should be construed by a consensus guideline statement by certifying boards.

SUMMARY

The steps involved in the placement of a permanent HBP lead fuse basic principles of EP with standard pacing lead implantation techniques. High-volume implanters with biventricular implanting experience will already have most of the skills required for mastering technical aspects of the procedure, with the complexity of the procedure lying in adapting skills associated with mapping and basic EP into the pacing realm. Although incorporating an EP target into permanent cardiac pacing increases the complexity of an otherwise routine process, there is a gratifying payoff with the prevention of iatrogenic dyssynchrony in patient with preserved HP function and the potential for true electrical resynchronization in patients with underlying HP disease.

As important as it is to focus on developing new skills required at the time of implant, it is equally important to educate device clinic personnel regarding the nuances of long-term HBP. There is some precedent for this type of transformation with the evolution of cardiac resynchronization therapy clinics. As the volume of His cases increase, it is critical to implement mechanisms for quality control and oversight to insure accurate threshold measurements and ideal His lead channel output throughout the patient's lifetime.

REFERENCES

1. Lustgarten DL, Crespo EM, Arkhipova-Jenkins I, et al. His-bundle pacing versus biventricular pacing in cardiac resynchronization therapy patients: a crossover design comparison. Heart Rhythm 2015;12(7):1548–57.

2. Vijayaraman P, Naperkowski A, Subzposh FA, et al. Permanent His-bundle pacing: long-term lead performance and clinical outcomes. Heart Rhythm 2018; 15(5):696–702.

3. Vijayaraman P, Dandamudi G, Zanon F, et al. Permanent His bundle pacing: recommendations from a multicenter His bundle pacing collaborative working group for standardization of definitions, implant measurements, and follow-up. Heart Rhythm 2018;15(3): 460–8.

4. Lustgarten DL. Step-wise approach to permanent His bundle pacing. JICRM 2016;7:2313–21.

5. Vijayaraman P, Dandamudi G, Worsnick S, et al. Acute His-bundle injury current during permanent his-bundle pacing predicts excellent pacing outcomes. Pacing Clin Electrophysiol 2015;38(5):540–6.

6. Lustgarten DL, Calame S, Crespo EM, et al. Electrical resynchronization induced by direct His-bundle pacing. Heart Rhythm 2010;7(1):15–21.

7. Narula OS. Longitudinal dissociation in the His bundle. Bundle branch block due to asynchronous conduction within the His bundle in man. Circulation 1977;56(6):996–1006.

How to Perform His Bundle Pacing: Tools and Techniques

Subodh Devabhaktuni, MD, Philip L. Mar, MD, Jonathan Shirazi, MD, Gopi Dandamudi, MD, FHRS*

KEYWORDS

- Pacemaker • Pacemaker implantation • Ventricular dyssynchrony • His bundle pacing
- Implantation technique • Device programming

KEY POINTS

- Permanent His bundle pacing (HBP) has been increasing in popularity as a pacing strategy in recent years.
- It offers true physiologic pacing with recruitment of the native Purkinje system, thereby preserving atrioventricular and interventricular synchrony.
- Careful attention to various responses to pacing (selective, nonselective, and septal) must be made to achieve long-term success.
- This form of pacing offers unique challenges to existing sensing and capture algorithms; newer pacing algorithms and technology will be required to achieve lasting success.

TOOLS AND TIPS FOR HIS BUNDLE PACING

His bundle pacing (HBP) has been gaining increasing recognition as a permanent pacing strategy in clinical practice. It offers true physiologic pacing, where both atrioventricular and interventricular/intraventricular synchrony are maintained. Performing HBP can be technically challenging for beginners because there is a learning curve, mostly because of limited tools in the setting of variable anatomies. With some experience, the authors think it can be performed in close to 90% of patients as shown in recent study.[1] By selecting the right patient and using the available tools appropriately, one can achieve the desired results in the vast majority of cases. The various tools necessary for the procedure include the following:

Pacing Lead

- 3830 Select Secure MRI SureScan His lead (Medtronic, Minneapolis, MN, USA) has a lead outer diameter of 4.2 F (French) with a 1.8-mm exposed and active helix (**Fig. 1**). It is a 69-cm-long solid core lead and requires the use of an outer sheath for placement.

Sheaths

There are 2 specific sheaths:

- C315 His sheath (Medtronic): It is a nondeflectable sheath with an inner diameter of 5.5 F and an outer diameter of 7.0 F (**Fig. 2**). It is 43 cm long with a primary curve to reach the superior aspect of the tricuspid annulus and a secondary curve to reach the septum.
- C304-69 sheath (Medtronic): It is a deflectable sheath with inner diameter of 5.7 F and an outer diameter of 8.4 F with unidirectional deflection (**Fig. 3**). It can be helpful in challenging anatomic situations, such as dilated right atria and an inferiorly displaced HB. Disadvantages, compared with the C315 His sheath, include lack of a secondary septal

Disclosures Statement: None (S. Devabhaktuni, P.L. Mar, J. Shirazi); Consultant & research support, Medtronic, Inc (G. Dandamudi).
Indiana University School of Medicine, Indianapolis, IN, USA
* Corresponding author. Indiana University School of Medicine, 1801 North Senate Boulevard, Indianapolis, IN 46202.
E-mail address: gdandamu@iu.edu

Card Electrophysiol Clin 10 (2018) 495–502
https://doi.org/10.1016/j.ccep.2018.05.008

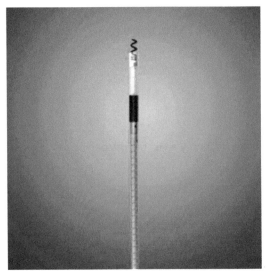

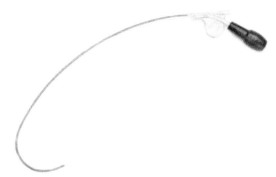

Fig. 3. C304-69 sheath (Medtronic): It is a deflectable sheath with inner diameter of 5.7 F and an outer diameter of 8.4 F with unidirectional deflection. Note the lack of a secondary septal curve. (*Courtesy of* Medtronic, Minneapolis, MN; with permission.)

Fig. 1. The 3830 Select Secure MRI SureScan His lead (Medtronic) has a lead outer diameter of 4.2 F with a 1.8-mm exposed and active helix. It is a solid core lead and requires the use of an outer sheath for placement. (*Reproduced with permission of* Medtronic, Inc.)

curve and difficulty stabilizing the lead as it is being screwed into the tissue.

A regular length 7 F peel-away sheath is used to place the His sheath through it. It allows for continued vascular access after the His sheath is split if needed.

ANALYZER

A pace-sense analyzer (PSA) is needed to record intracardiac electrograms (EGMs). The authors normally connect the pacing lead to the atrial channel of the Medtronic PSA because of the inherent sensing algorithms built into it. They use a higher gain setting of 0.05 mV/mm. For PSAs of other manufacturers, the lead is

connected to the ventricular channel. Also, while assessing for His bundle recordings, the highest sweep speed possible should be used to better assess the local EGMs (**Fig. 4**).

ELECTROPHYSIOLOGY RECORDING SYSTEM

Even though during their early implant experience the authors relied on the PSA alone to perform the procedure, they have been using the electrophysiology (EP) recording system available in EP laboratories to perform the procedure. Connections can be made to record the local EGMs from the lead tip simultaneously on the PSA as well as the EP recording systems. Advantages include the ability to adjust filter and gain settings to better delineate the His bundle EGMs and also the ability to assess for selective versus nonselective His bundle pacing (N-HBP) based on the local evoked responses to pacing (**Figs. 5** and **6**).

MAPPING CATHETER (AS NEEDED)

Historically, an EP mapping catheter was routinely used to locate the HB. However, the authors routinely use the pacing lead to map the HB. If needed, the mapping catheter can be advanced from above. The use of a mapping catheter can be helpful where concomitant atrioventricular junction ablation and HBP are being performed. The His bundle EGMs can be marked with the ablation catheter (His cloud) before placing the lead.

Unipolar mapping technique is used during initial mapping with the pacing lead as the proximal pole is often inside the sheath to provide lead stability.

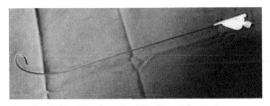

Fig. 2. C315 His sheath (Medtronic): It is a nondeflectable sheath with an inner diameter of 5.5 F and an outer diameter of 7.0 F. It is 43 cm long with a primary curve to reach the superior aspect of the tricuspid annulus and a secondary curve to reach the septum. (*Reproduced with permission of* Medtronic, Inc.)

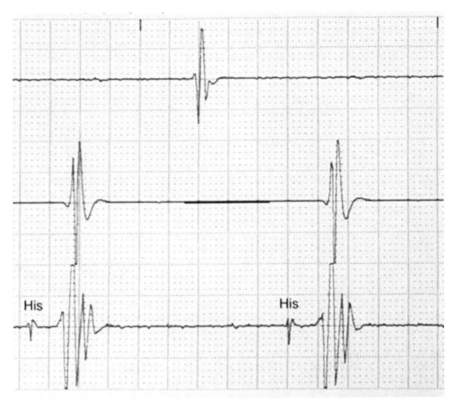

Fig. 4. Bipolar EGMs from the pacing lead recorded on the PSA during a pacemaker implant. Note the clear His bundle EGMs that can be seen using the PSA.

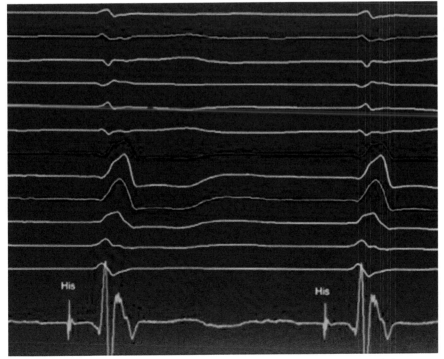

Fig. 5. Unipolar EGMs from the pacing lead recorded using the EP recording system. High-frequency His bundle EGMs can be clearly recorded in this case. The patient has underlying RBB block and a prolonged HV interval.

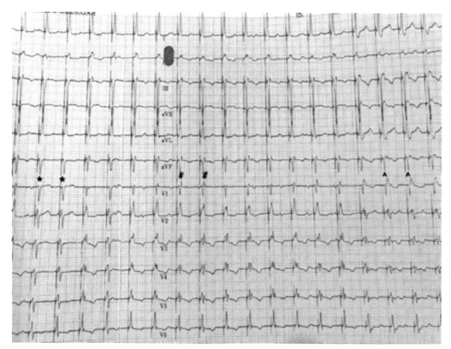

Fig. 6. Pacing output is gradually reduced from left to right during HBP. This example highlights the importance of using a 12-lead ECG in assessing responses to changes in pacing output. Asterisk, selective HBP; hash, selective HBP with partial recruitment of the RBB; caret, selective HBP with loss of RBB recruitment.

12-LEAD ELECTROCARDIOGRAM

One of the most important aspects of this procedure is to use a 12-lead electrocardiographic (ECG) recording during the case. Subtle differences can differentiate pacing-HBP versus septal pacing on certain occasions, and the 12-lead ECG allows for such discrimination. This point cannot be overemphasized when performing permanent HBP.

IMPLANT TECHNIQUE

Once vascular access is obtained (cephalic, axillary, or subclavian vein), a guidewire is advanced into the right atrium (RA) or right ventricle (RV). A 7-F sheath can be advanced over the wire to retain access. Otherwise, the C315 His sheath is advanced into the RA or RV and the guidewire is removed. The sheath usually tends to settle toward the anterior/superior tricuspid annulus near the HB region. Thereafter, the pacing lead is advanced to the tip of the sheath, with the distal tip of the lead exposed minimally. Unipolar connections are made with the tip of the lead and tissue. Clockwise rotation allows for more anterior movement toward the ventricle, and counterclockwise rotation allows for more posterior movement within the RA. Typically, from

the RA, gentle clockwise rotation is applied to reach the septum in close proximity to the tricuspid annulus. If large RV EGMs are noted, the apparatus is gently pulled back to the atrioventricular grove with minimal counterclockwise rotation to ensure that the lead tip is abutting the septum. Once an atrial to ventricular EGMs ratio of 1:2 or greater is noted, the sheath is pointed toward the superior-anterior septum or midposterior septum by minimal clockwise or counterclockwise rotation, respectively. Small movements are encouraged because HB deflections can be easily missed. It is crucial to maneuver the lead to achieve a high-frequency near-field HB recording because this indicates that the lead tip is in good contact with the septum. If low-frequency far-field HB EGMs are recorded, this usually indicates poor contact with the septum.

It is also important for both the operator and the person operating the PSA/EP recording system to pay careful attention to intracardiac EGMs. The authors usually set the sweep speed to 50 or 100 mm/s to allow better separation of atrial, HB, and local ventricular EGMs and gain settings of 0.05 mV/mm. Once HB EGMs are obtained, unipolar pacing is performed because the proximal pole of the lead is within the sheath. The authors start pacing at 5 V at 1 millisecond and assess 12-lead

QRS morphologies. The following responses can be observed:

A. Selective HB pacing (S-HBP): Stimulus to ventricular activation is equal to the intrinsic HV interval and paced QRS morphology is identical to the intrinsic narrow QRS complex. Sometimes, S-HBP can occur without either left bundle branch (LBB) or right bundle branch (RBB) recruitment (see **Fig. 6**).

B. Non-selective HB pacing (NS-HBP): Stimulus-ventricular activation is shorter than the HV interval and there is local fusion with capture of both HB and local septal myocardium (**Fig. 7**). Pacing output is decremented to assess the changing QRS morphologies to differentiate NS-HBP from RV septal pacing.

With NS-HBP, different patterns may be observed:

1. At higher output, the HB is preferentially recruited with progressive widening as output is reduced, resulting in more local ventricular capture (similar to para-hisian pacing performed to assess for septal accessory pathways).
2. At higher output, more fusion is encountered because of local ventricular capture, and at lower output, HB is preferentially activated, resulting in less fusion.
3. On some occasions, pure HBP can be seen just before loss of capture. Also, selective RBB or LBB conduction can be demonstrated.
4. On some occasions, because of the proximity of RBB and more ventricular placement of the lead, RBB capture can occur resulting in a LBB block pattern QRS complex. It may be difficult to determine whether local myocardial

capture occurs along with RBB capture. If intrinsic conduction is present, measuring the HV interval can help determine RBB capture. Typically, a local HV interval would be short (<30 milliseconds), with no far field atrial EGM seen on the PSA.

Thereafter, once the HB location is identified, the fluoroscopic image is saved as a reference. The sheath is held steady by the left hand, and the pacing lead is slowly rotated clockwise approximately 5 times. It is important to ensure that the lead torque is transmitted to the tip of the lead. With adequate torque buildup, the lead usually rotates back counterclockwise if the lead is anchored well to the HB region. The sheath is pulled back while the lead is gently held forward until a loop is formed in the atrium. After the lead is screwed in, His bundle injury current can be demonstrated in approximately 40% of patients[2] (**Fig. 8**). The injury current may merge with the local ventricular EGM. It has been previously shown that the presence of His bundle injury current at implant is associated with lower His capture thresholds compared with those without demonstrable injury current.[3] Testing is performed in both unipolar and bipolar configurations. Starting at 5 V at 1 millisecond, output is decremented to assess response to pacing. Either selective or nonselective HBP is accepted, and pacing thresholds less than 2 V at 1 millisecond are generally considered acceptable. If the patient is pacemaker dependent, lower pacing thresholds along with NS-HBP (fusion due to local septal capture serves as a backup) are desirable before accepting the final lead position. If the pacing threshold margins

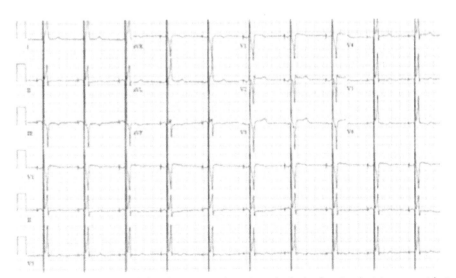

Fig. 7. N- HBP in a patient with a dual chamber pacemaker. Note the lack of an isoelectric segment between the stimulus artifact and the QRS onset and also fusion with septal capture within the first 40 milliseconds of pacing.

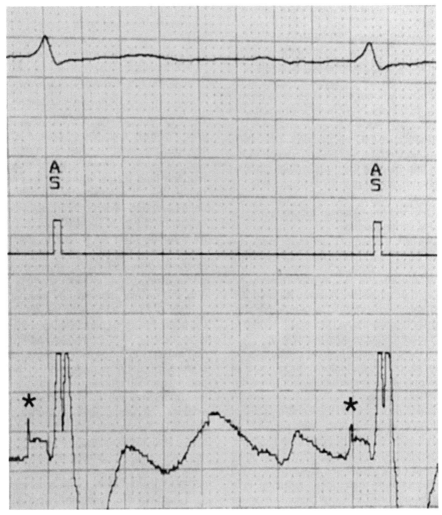

Fig. 8. Unipolar EGMs recorded from the pacing lead using the PSA. Asterisk, acute His bundle current of injury.

are not at or below the acceptable value after multiple attempts, the lead can be placed slightly anteriorly, resulting in RV septal pacing. The authors monitor the patient overnight on telemetry, and the device system is interrogated the next day before discharge.

TROUBLESHOOTING
His-Bundle Localization and Fixation Mechanisms

One of the challenging issues that first-time implanters have is difficulty with His bundle localization and subsequent attachment of the pacing lead. Unlike placement of an EP catheter, the lead tip surface area is relatively small and it lies perpendicular to the septum. Care must be taken to gently move the lead and sheath apparatus along the septum close to the annulus. The

cardiac fat pad near the coronary sinus can be used as a reference. In this regard, the use of the C315 His sheath, which has a curve that naturally directs the pacing lead toward the atrial septum near the tricuspid annulus, can result in early identification of the His bundle in 80% of cases.[4] The secondary septal curve of the C315 also provides a more perpendicular configuration with the surface of the atrial septum, allowing better force alignment to screw in the pacing lead.[2]

For challenging cases where it is difficult to locate His EGMs with the C315 His sheath, the C304 His sheath can be used. However, because of lack of a septal curve, lead fixation can be challenging at times. Another technique that can be used is to use a coronary sinus guiding catheter. This sheath can be cut at the hub and used as an outer guiding catheter to provide more support and lift to reach the superior aspect of the septum (**Fig. 9**).

In dependent patients with no intrinsic rhythm, careful pace-mapping can be used to assess His bundle capture based on 12-lead morphology.

Sensing Issues

After fixation of the lead onto the septum near the tricuspid annulus, the atrial EGM at the tip is usually much smaller than the ventricular EGM. Therefore, atrial oversensing is usually not an issue. Occasionally, far-field atrial EGMs can be large enough to be oversensed on the ventricular channel. Care must be taken to avoid this phenomenon because ventricular pacing may be inhibited. Also, occasionally, large His bundle EGMs can be oversensed on the ventricular channel as well. Sensing on the ventricular channel can be variable as well.

With S-HBP, sensing can be as low as 1 mV, and once again, care must be taken to ensure that there is no atrial oversensing or ventricular undersensing. Devices can have separate ceilings for ventricular sensing, and this needs to be kept in mind when the proper pulse generator is being selected (ie, Medtronic Sensia >1.2 mV vs Medtronic Advisa >0.3 mV). Sometimes unipolar sensing allows for better discrimination, and in nondependent patients, it can be used to offer better sensing safety margins.[2] Long-term issues with oversensing and undersensing are rare, occurring in less than 1% patients, and highlight the importance of achieving optimal sensing parameters at implantation.[4] Furthermore, in certain situations where only a single lead needs to be implanted (chronic atrial fibrillation), the maximal sensitivity settings for certain pacing modes can be exploited, such as using AAI mode (sensitivity 0.15 mV) versus VVI mode (sensitivity 1 mV).[4]

Pacing Issues: Capture Threshold and Optimization of Battery Life

One of the biggest concerns with HBP is the higher pacing thresholds compared with conventional RV pacing, which can result in earlier battery depletion than desired. Typically, higher pacing thresholds occur in less than 10% of patients during the first 3 months and are thought to be related to microdislodgement and local fibrosis.[4] Although acute thresholds may increase, chronic thresholds tend to be stable. An initial capture threshold of less than 2 V at 1 millisecond during implantation will usually result in durable and persistent capture thresholds. The demonstration of a His bundle injury current with initial fixation of the pacing lead is also prognostic for lower and more durable long-term pacing thresholds.[3]

The device with the largest battery capacity within a manufacturer's pacemaker service line is chosen during implantation. To prolong the longevity of a device, the pulse width is increased to 1 millisecond so that the amplitude can be decreased. In dependent patients with S-HBP and high capture thresholds, an RV lead can be implanted for backup pacing only so that the HBP outputs can be decreased to the lowest threshold possible without fear of intermittent noncapture.[4] The automatic threshold testing algorithms should not be used because of their inability to accurately detect true His capture.[2]

FOLLOW-UP

Unlike traditional pacing, HBP requires more intense follow-up in the first 3 to 6 months. Ideally, all patients should be discharged home on remote

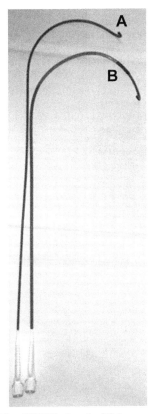

Fig. 9. (*A*) The C315 His sheath. (*B*) A composite of the Attain command multipurpose guiding catheter and the C315 His sheath. In this case, the multipurpose catheter is cut a few centimeters from the hub and advanced over the C315 His sheath. This apparatus can then be gently shaped to create a larger curve with a telescoping mechanism. This allows for better reach in a dilated RA (all sheaths are made by Medtronic). (*Reproduced with permission of Medtronic, Inc.*)

monitoring. Postprocedure follow-up should be established within a few weeks, and a 12-lead ECG rhythm strip is important to document when true HB capture is lost. Detailing proper responses allows for programming of adequate safety margins while optimizing batter performance. It is very important that the device clinic nurses and device company technicians are educated on the nuances of HBP and are able to recognize subtle issues that can lead to long-term complications if not properly addressed. In the authors' practice, it is customary for the implanting physician to see the patient at 2 weeks' and 3 months' follow-up, respectively.

SUMMARY

Permanent HBP has emerged as a viable pacing strategy in routine clinical practice. It allows for true physiologic pacing by using the native His Purkinje system and avoiding the deleterious effects of chronic right ventricular pacing. In its current form, success rates are anywhere from 80% to 90%. As the understanding and technology improve, it is likely to achieve a stronger foothold as a common strategy for chronic ventricular pacing.

REFERENCES

1. Sharma PS, Dandamudi G, Herweg B, et al. Permanent His-bundle pacing as an alternative to biventricular pacing for cardiac resynchronization therapy: a multicenter experience. Heart Rhythm 2018;15(3):413–20.

2. Vijayaraman P, Dandamudi G. How to perform permanent his bundle pacing: tips and tricks. Pacing Clin Electrophysiol 2016;39:1298–304.

3. Vijayaraman P, Dandamudi G, Worsnick S, et al. Acute his-bundle injury current during permanent his-bundle pacing predicts excellent pacing outcomes. Pacing Clin Electrophysiol 2015;38:540–6.

4. Dandamudi G, Vijayaraman P. How to perform permanent His bundle pacing in routine clinical practice. Heart Rhythm 2016;13:1362–6.

Hemodynamics of His Bundle Pacing

Amrish Deshmukh, MD[a], Umashankar Lakshmanadoss, MD[b], Pramod Deshmukh, MD[c],*

KEYWORDS

- Hemodynamics • Septal pacing • Apical pacing • His bundle pacing

KEY POINTS

- Hemodynamic studies have demonstrated that right ventricular apical pacing leads to abnormal electromechanical ventricular activation and impaired hemodynamic parameters in comparison with intrinsic conduction.
- His bundle pacing and septal pacing have been demonstrated to have superior hemodynamics to right ventricular apical pacing.
- This article provides data that demonstrate a superior hemodynamic profile with His bundle pacing in comparison with septal and apical pacing.

INTRODUCTION

The His–Purkinje conduction system ensures a rapid coordinated multisite activation of the ventricles. The potential for artificial pacing to alter this activation sequence and thereby impair ventricular contractile function was first described by Wiggers in 1925.[1] Despite this knowledge, the right ventricular (RV) apex became established as the default site of implantation for ventricular pacemakers owing to technological limitations and convenience. During this experience, chronic RV apical pacing (RVAP) has been associated with the development of cardiomyopathy, incident atrial fibrillation, and heart failure hospitalization.[2–7] With the advent of active fixation leads, numerous alternative sites of pacing within the RV, RV outflow tract (RVOT), and conduction system have been investigated to recapitulate the physiologic activation of the ventricles.[8–11] This article summarizes investigations comparing the hemodynamics of direct His bundle pacing (DHBP) with RVAP and septal pacing.

VENTRICULAR ACTIVATION AND CONTRACTION WITH RIGHT VENTRICULAR APICAL PACING

In contrast with the rapid and synchronous activation of the ventricles coordinated by the His–Purkinje system, ventricular activation with RVAP proceeds by slow and heterogeneous myocardial conduction resulting in interventricular and intraventricular dyssynchrony in excitation and contraction. Similar to left bundle branch block, RVAP produces prolonged left ventricular (LV) activation and results in latest activation of the inferoposterior base.[12] However, in contrast with left bundle branch block, RVAP also further prolongs RV excitation and leads to greater differences in the activation times of the right and left ventricles.[13] The resulting impairment in ventricular function was first investigated by Badke and colleagues,[14] who found mechanical dyssynchrony in parallel with electrical dyssynchrony. Contraction in the septum and earlier activated regions of the ventricle with RVAP-induced stretch of late activated regions before peak systole. In

Disclosure: This research was financially supported, in part, by Medtronic.
[a] Department of Medicine, University of Chicago, 5841 South Maryland Avenue, MC 6092, Chicago, IL 60637, USA; [b] Cardiac Electrophysiology Division, Ballad Health CVA Heart Institute, 2050 Meadowview Pkwy, Kingsport, TN 37660, USA; [c] Cardiac and Vascular Center, Arrhythmia Center, Robert Packer Hospital, 1 Guthrie Square, Sayre, PA 18840, USA
* Corresponding author.
E-mail address: prmode@yahoo.com

addition, late activated regions demonstrated delayed shortening, which continued into early diastole. The global consequence of these segmental derangements was a decreased peak systolic pressure and rate of LV pressure increase (dP/dt) with RVAP.[14] This abnormal pattern of activation was confirmed by subsequent studies, which also demonstrated increased myofiber work in late activated regions, increased myocardial oxygen consumption, asymmetric hypertrophy, and ventricular dilation.[2,15,16]

HEMODYNAMICS OF HIS BUNDLE PACING
Comparison of His Bundle Pacing and Right Ventricular Apical Pacing

DHBP has been compared directly with RVAP by several authors. In an intrapatient study of 23 patients, Catanzariti and colleagues[17] found that, in comparison with DHBP, RVAP was associated with greater echocardiographic interventricular dyssynchrony, increased echocardiographic intraventricular dyssynchrony, and a worsened Tei index. Kronborg and colleagues[18] demonstrated that, compared with DHBP, RVAP resulted in prolonged time to peak velocity between basal segments by tissue Doppler ultrasound examination and lower LV outflow tract velocity time integral. In a later study, Catanzariti and colleagues[19] found an increased interventricular conduction delay, increased mechanical dyssynchrony, increased mitral regurgitation, and decreased LV ejection fraction with RVAP.

Comparison of Septal Pacing and Right Ventricular Apical Pacing

In addition to the His bundle, numerous other sites have been evaluated as alternatives to RVAP. Of these selective sites, the best characterized are the septal aspect of the RV and RVOT. Initial short-term and hemodynamic studies demonstrated that, compared with RVAP, RVOT and RV septal pacing resulted in narrower QRS, higher cardiac indices, increased dP/dt, and increased ejection fraction.[9,20–22] Similarly, in -term follow-up studies, in comparison with RVAP, RVOT and septal pacing were associated with improved ejection fraction and improved indices of ventricular synchrony.[10,23–25]

Comparison of His Bundle Pacing, Septal Pacing, and Right Ventricular Apical Pacing

Few reported studies have compared the acute hemodynamics of His bundle pacing, RVOT and RV septal pacing, and RVAP. Here we present a small intrapatient comparison from our group.

Methods
Seven patients (5 males and 2 females) with chronic atrial fibrillation and heart failure with reduced ejection fraction underwent atrioventricular nodal ablation and permanent His bundle pacemaker implantation. Clinical characteristics of the patients are presented in **Table 1**. All patients had a QRS duration of less than 120 milliseconds. All patients provided written informed consent according to a protocol approved by the Institutional Review Board of Guthrie Health System.

Hemodynamic evaluation Hemodynamic evaluation was performed using 6-F high-resolution pressure sensing catheters (Mikro-tip model SVPC-664D, Millar Instruments, Inc., Houston, TX) in the RV and LV. Pressure transducers were connected to a Bio-Tek DPM-IB pneumatic transducer tester (Bio-Tek Instruments Inc, Winooski, VT). Signals were processed, sampled at 512 Hz and archived using LabVIEW (National Instruments Inc, Austin, TX). LV and RV hemodynamic measurements included the maximum rate of LV and RV pressure increase (dP/dt_{max}) and decrease (dP/dt_{min}).

Table 1
Patient characteristics

Patient	Gender	Age (y)	Weight (lbs)	NYHA Functional Class	LVEF (%)	Cardiovascular History
1	M	78	200	2	30	DCM, HTN, CABG
2	F	69	124	3	30	DCM, HTN, MVR
3	M	60	240	2	45	DCM, CAD, COPD
4	M	61	175	3	30	DCM, CAD
5	F	62	190	2	30	DCM, CAD, COPD
6	M	64	199	3	20	DCM, CAD, COPD,
7	M	80	267	3	30	DCM, CAD, HTN

Abbreviations: CABG, coronary artery bypass graft; CAD, coronary artery disease; COPD, chronic obstructive pulmonary disease; DCM, dilated cardiomyopathy; HTN, hypertension; MVR, mitral valve replacement; NYHA, New York Heart Association.

Pacing sites and protocol The effects of ventricular pacing were evaluated from 4 sites: His bundle (DHBP), high RV septum (high RVS), low RV septum (low RVS), and RV apex (RVAP). Multiple fluoroscopic projections and electrocardiograms were used to confirm lead position. RV septal pacing was confirmed via lead I with initially negative isoelectric deflection. Pacing in the high RVS was confirmed more positive QRS deflection in leads II, II and aVF when compared with the low RVS. DHBP and RVAP were achieved using the preexistent pacemaker. A Bloom EP stimulator (Fisher Medical Technologies, Inc., Wheat Ridge, CO) was used otherwise. Pacing was tested at each site for a duration of 4 minutes at a rate of 60, 80, 100, and 120 bpm.

Data analysis The impact of pacing site on LV and RV hemodynamic function was determined using MATLAB (MathWorks Inc, Natick, MA). Hemodynamic indices measured at various site and rate combinations were analyzed using analysis of variance with repeated measures and multiple comparison testing. LV and RV hemodynamics were compared by normalizing dP/dt_{max} at each site at 80, 100, and 120 bpm to dP/dt_{max} during DHBP at 60 bpm (ie, baseline) with a subsequent application of analysis of variance with repeated measures and interaction testing. Finally, comparisons of QRS durations and electrical axes obtained from each site during pacing at 60 bpm were made using repeated measures analysis of variance with multiple comparisons.

Results
A total of 7 patients (71% male; mean age, 68 ± 8 years; New York Heart Association functional class 2.6 ± 0.5; 85% with coronary artery disease; 71% with hypertension; 28% with diabetes mellitus; and 14% with coronary artery bypass graft) with chronic atrial fibrillation (45 ± 9 months) and reduced LV ejection fraction (30.7 ± 7.3) who underwent an atrioventricular nodal ablation and permanent DHBP pacemaker insertion were included (see **Table 1**).

Impact of pacing site on electrical axis and QRS duration
QRS axes viewed from the frontal plane were normal during DHBP, high and low RVS pacing but deviated to the left with RVAP pacing. High RVS and low RVS pacing resulted in a rightward shift of the QRS axis within the normal range. As expected, RVAP pacing resulted in pronounced left axis deviation. Mean QRS duration was relatively normal during DHBP, but significantly widened at all RV paced sites ($P<.05$; **Fig. 1, Table 2**).

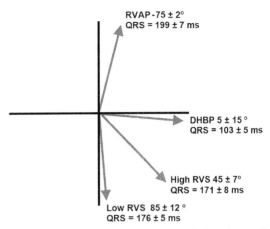

Fig. 1. Frontal plane QRS axes and durations of different pacing modes. DHBP, direct His bundle pacing; RVAP, right ventricular apical pacing; RVS, right ventricular septum.

Effect of pacing site and rate on left ventricular performance
Normal ventricular activation via DHBP at 60 and 80 bpm produced LV dP/dt_{max} that was significantly higher than during low RVS and RVAP ($P<.05$), yet comparable with high RVS pacing. LV dP/dt_{max} during DHBP at 100 bpm was higher than all RV sites ($P<.05$), but no significant difference was seen across pacing sites at 120 bpm (**Fig. 2**). Detectable differences in LV relaxation rate (ie, dP/dt_{min}) were seen during DHBP at 60, 80, and 100 bpm compared with RV sites ($P<.05$; **Table 3**).

Increasing the pacing rate contributed to a significant increase in LV dP/dt_{max} for all pacing sites. Peak diastolic relaxation rate (ie, dP/dt_{min}) trended higher with increased pacing rate for DHBP and high RVS sites but lacked statistical significance. LV end-systolic pressure (ESP) trended toward lower values with increased pacing rate for all sites except RVA, from which pacing significantly

Table 2
Mean ECG axes and QRS widths during pacing from different sites

Pacing Site	DHBP	High RVS	Low RVS	RVAP
QRS duration (ms)	103 ± 5*	171 ± 8	176 ± 5	199 ± 7
QRS axis	5 ± 15°	45 ± 7°	85 ± 12°	−75 ± 2°

Abbreviations: DHBP, direct His bundle pacing; RVAP, right ventricular apical pacing; RVS, right ventricular septum.
° is used to indicate degrees as a unit of measurement in all tables and figures.
* indicates $P<.05$ for comparison of groups in one way ANOVA.

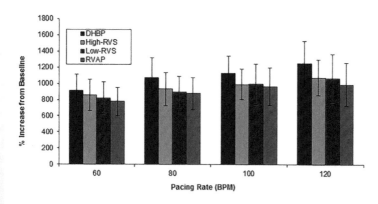

Fig. 2. Differences in left ventricular decreased peak systolic pressure and rate of left ventricular pressure increase at different pacing sites and rates. DHBP, direct His bundle pacing; RVAP, right ventricular apical pacing; RVS, right ventricular septum.

increased LVESP at 100 bpm ($P<.05$). Similarly, low RVS pacing at 120 bpm resulted in a significant decrease in LVESP compared with 80 and 100 bpm ($P<.05$). A significant decrease in the LV end-diastolic pressure (EDP) at increased pacing rates of 100 and 120 bpm was observed only during DHBP and during low RVS pacing at 120 bpm ($P<.05$; see **Table 3**; **Table 4**).

Table 3
LV and RV dP/dt$_{max}$ and dP/dt$_{min}$ during DHBP, high RVS, low RVS, and RVAP

	LV (mm Hg/s)		RV (mm Hg/s)	
	dP/dt$_{max}$	dP/dt$_{min}$	dP/dt$_{max}$	dP/dt$_{min}$
DHBP				
60	912 ± 198[a]	−1058 ± 133[b,c]	316 ± 98	−282 ± 85
80	1077 ± 244[a]	−1191 ± 213[c]	382 ± 143	−309 ± 89
100	1128 ± 217[d,e]	−1218 ± 211[c]	384 ± 158	−281 ± 70
120	1250 ± 280[d]	−1188 ± 285	420 ± 159[f]	−286 ± 91
High RVS				
60	860 ± 193	−912 ± 96	277 ± 97	−262 ± 53
80	932 ± 205	−980 ± 104	377 ± 97	−269 ± 55
100	992 ± 189[d]	−1024 ± 156	375 ± 86[d]	−254 ± 49
120	1075 ± 219[d,g]	−1011 ± 220	378 ± 93[d]	−256 ± 78
Low RVS				
60	823 ± 197	−947 ± 155	314 ± 115	−256 ± 62
80	896 ± 190	−1002 ± 123	370 ± 162	−258 ± 70
100	993 ± 249[d]	−1027 ± 189	407 ± 172[d]	−261 ± 73
120	1069 ± 295[d,g]	−984 ± 237	452 ± 194[d,g]	−257 ± 81
RVAP				
60	777 ± 173	−1009 ± 159	278 ± 81	−265 ± 92
80	879 ± 196	−1058 ± 209	334 ± 120	−300 ± 110
100	966 ± 228[d]	−1039 ± 167	346 ± 132	−274 ± 97
120	992 ± 266[d]	−986 ± 227	377 ± 130	−273 ± 122

Abbreviations: dP/dt$_{max}$, maximum rate of left ventricular and right ventricular pressure increase; dP/dt$_{min}$, minimum rate of left ventricular and right ventricular pressure increase; DHBP, direct His bundle pacing; LV, left ventricular; RV, right ventricular; RVAP, right ventricular apical pacing; RVS, right ventricular septum.
 [a] $P<.05$; LV dP/dt$_{max}$: DHBP 60 and 80 bpm versus low RVS and RVAP.
 [b] $P<.05$; LV dP/dt$_{min}$: DHBP 60 bpm versus 100 bpm.
 [c] $P<.05$; LV dP/dt$_{min}$: DHBP 60, 80, and 100 bpm versus high RVS, low RVS.
 [d] $P<.05$; LV dP/dt$_{max}$; All sites at 100 and 120 bpm versus RVAP and low RVS at 60 bpm.
 [e] $P<.05$; LV dP/dt$_{max}$: DHBP 100 bpm versus high RVS, low RVS and RVAP.
 [f] $P<.05$; RV dP/dt$_{max}$; DHBP at 120 bpm versus RVAP and Low RVS at 60 bpm.
 [g] $P<.05$; LV and RV dP/dt$_{max}$; high RVS and low RVS 60 bpm versus 120 bpm.

Table 4
LV and RV end-diastolic pressure and peak systolic pressure following DHBP, high RVS, low RVS, and RVAP

Pacing Site	Pacing Rate (bpm)	LV		RV	
		EDP	ESP	EDP	ESP
DHBP	60	14.8 ± 8.9	105.0 ± 21.1	12.2 ± 8.1	41.3 ± 8.1
	80	13.3 ± 7.3	113.3 ± 16.9	8.8 ± 6.7	40.5 ± 6.8
	100	12.1 ± 8.0^a	107.6 ± 16.0	10.5 ± 9.6	38.0 ± 9.8
	120	9.9 ± 8.4^a	99.5 ± 11.6	10.6 ± 9.6	37.0 ± 9.5
High RVS	60	13.7 ± 6.7	95.4 ± 11.6	10.9 ± 7.2	41.2 ± 7.2
	80	11.9 ± 6.5	97.7 ± 12.9	10.9 ± 7.2	39.6 ± 4.9
	100	10.1 ± 6.1	95.8 ± 11.6	10.2 ± 9.1	36.2 ± 8.3
	120	9.2 ± 6.0	90.6 ± 14.9	9.4 ± 7.3	34.0 ± 7.2
Low RVS	60	16.0 ± 5.9	101.4 ± 16.2	15.5 ± 6.1	44.9 ± 4.7
	80	14.7 ± 6.9	104.4 ± 15.3	14.1 ± 7.2	42.7 ± 5.3
	100	14.3 ± 7.0	103.5 ± 17.7	14.0 ± 8.4	41.2 ± 6.8
	120	12.8 ± 7.0^b	95.1 ± 22.0	13.8 ± 8.2	39.6 ± 8.4^c
RVAP	60	14.7 ± 8.2	97.7 ± 17.7	14.4 ± 7.8	43.4 ± 5.7
	80	13.8 ± 6.0	102.2 ± 13.7	13.4 ± 6.9	41.4 ± 4.4
	100	12.3 ± 7.9	98.0 ± 18.8	12.2 ± 8.6^d	37.2 ± 8.3^a
	120	11.4 ± 7.6	91.6 ± 22.4^e	12.7 ± 9.5	37.0 ± 9.2^a

Abbreviations: DHBP, direct His bundle pacing; LV, left ventricular; RV, right ventricular; RVAP, right ventricular apical pacing; RVS, right ventricular septum.

[a] $P<.05$; LVEDP; 60 bpm versus 100 and 120 bpm, RVESP 60 bpm versus 100 and 120 bpm.
[b] $P<.05$; LVEDP 60 bpm versus 120 bpm.
[c] $P<.05$; RVESP; 80 bpm and 100 vs 120 bpm.
[d] $P<.05$; RVEDP; 60 bpm versus 100 bpm.
[e] $P<.05$; LVESP; 80 bpm versus 120 bpm.

Effect of pacing site and rate on right ventricular performance

RV hemodynamic indices were not influenced by pacing site; however, rate effects were observed. DHBP pacing at 120 bpm generated RV dP/dt_{max} values that were significantly higher than at 60 bpm ($P<.05$). Significant increases in RV dP/dt_{max} were also observed at increased heart rates during low RVS and RVAP, but not during high RVS pacing. RV ESP was unaffected by pacing rate during DHBP, high RVS, and low RVS pacing, yet a significant decrease in RV ESP at increased rates of 100 and 120 bpm occurred during RVAP. Similarly, RV EDP was unaltered with increased heart rate during DHBP, high RVS, or low RVS pacing. A significant decrease in RV EDP was observed with only with RVAP at 100 bpm ($P<.05$; see **Tables 3** and **4**).

Effect of pacing site and rate on biventricular performance

When comparing the contractile response between the LV and RV for each pacing site, DHBP achieved the greatest relative increases in LV and RV dP/dt_{max} or force–frequency relationship. The LV force–frequency relationship response was comparable with that of the RV force–frequency relationship during DHBP. At all other sites, the force–frequency relationship response was more pronounced in the RV compared with the LV (**Fig. 3**; see **Table 3**).

Discussion

These results demonstrate superior hemodynamic performance with DHBP as a result of physiologic stimulation of the His–Purkinje system as compared with other septal pacing sites and RVAP. Specifically, the finding that DHBP significantly increased the LV dP/dt_{max} with a maintained EDP and ESP indicates increased LV inotropy. With regard to LV relaxation, highest dP/dt_{min} with DHBP provides evidence of improved lusitropy, particularly during isovolumetric relaxation. Finally, DHBP demonstrates concordant RV and LV force–frequency relationship with increased pacing rates in contrast to other RV pacing sites.

Discrepant findings by a similar study by Padeletti and colleagues[26] in 2007 were likely due to differences in methods and patient characteristics. This study compared the effect of RV pacing site on LV hemodynamic performance in 12 humans with intact AV conduction and demonstrated no improvement in LV dP/dt_{max}, LV ESP, LV

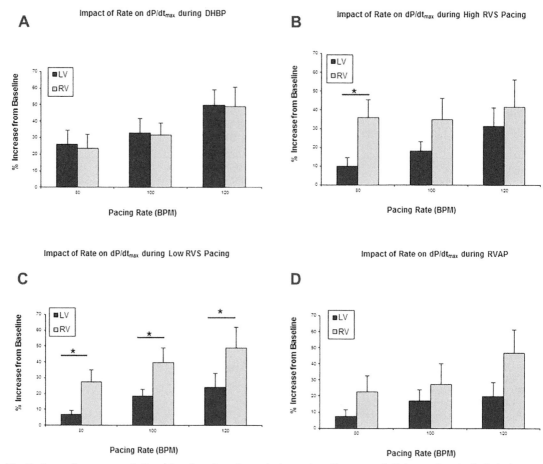

Fig. 3. Force–frequency relationship of pacing sites relative to baseline rate of 60 bpm. Sites included *A*) DHBP *B*) High RVS *C*) Low RVS *D*) RVAP. In comparison with other sites of right ventricular pacing, DHBP (*A*) demonstrates a concordant force–frequency relationship in the left and right ventricles relative to the baseline pacing rate of 60 beats per minute (*BPM*). dP/dtmax, maximum left ventricular decreased peak systolic pressure and rate of left ventricular pressure increase. * indicates $P<.05$ for t-test for group comparisons. LV, left ventricle; RV, right ventricle; RVAP, right ventricular apical pacing; RVS, right ventricular septum.

EDP, or cycle efficiency during DHBP compared with atrial-triggered RV septal pacing and RVAP. These differences are likely attributable to the likelihood of bimodal (ie, fused) ventricular activation during atrial synchronous RV septal pacing and RVAP in patients with normal AV conduction. The heterogeneity of the patient group compared with our study may also account for the differences with 25% of patients having a QRS duration of greater than 120 ms.

SUMMARY

DHBP preserves the native electromechanical activation of the ventricles and in numerous studies demonstrates improved hemodynamic parameters relative to RVAP. Alternative RV pacing sites, including the septal RV, may more closely approximate physiologic ventricular activation and in some long-term studies show benefit relative to RVAP. In our acute study, DHBP demonstrates superior hemodynamic parameters relative to RV septal pacing and RVAP. Longer term and larger studies are needed to elucidate whether DHBP provides a benefit relative to RV septal pacing or indirect His bundle pacing.

REFERENCES

1. Wiggers CJ. The muscular reactions of the mammalian ventricles to artificial surface stimuli. Am J Physiol 1925;73(2):346–78.
2. van Oosterhout MF, Prinzen FW, Arts T, et al. Asynchronous electrical activation induces asymmetrical hypertrophy of the left ventricular wall. Circulation 1998;98(6):588–95.

3. Andersen HR, Nielsen JC, Thomsen PE, et al. Long-term follow-up of patients from a randomised trial of atrial versus ventricular pacing for sick-sinus syndrome. Lancet 1997;350(9086):1210–6.

4. Connolly SJ, Kerr CR, Gent M, et al. Effects of physiologic pacing versus ventricular pacing on the risk of stroke and death due to cardiovascular causes. N Engl J Med 2000;342(19):1385–91.

5. Lamas GA, Lee KL, Sweeney MO, et al. Ventricular pacing or dual-chamber pacing for sinus-node dysfunction. N Engl J Med 2002;346(24):1854–62.

6. Wilkoff BL, Cook JR, Epstein AE, et al. Dual-chamber pacing or ventricular backup pacing in patients with an implantable defibrillator: the Dual Chamber and VVI Implantable Defibrillator (DAVID) Trial. JAMA 2002;288(24):3115–23.

7. Sweeney MO, Hellkamp AS, Ellenbogen KA, et al. Adverse effect of ventricular pacing on heart failure and atrial fibrillation among patients with normal baseline QRS duration in a clinical trial of pacemaker therapy for sinus node dysfunction. Circulation 2003;107(23):2932–7.

8. Deshmukh P, Casavant DA, Romanyshyn M, et al. Permanent, direct his-bundle pacing: a novel approach to cardiac pacing in patients with normal His-Purkinje activation. Circulation 2000;101(8): 869–77.

9. Victor F, Leclercq C, Mabo P, et al. Optimal right ventricular pacing site in chronically implanted patients: a prospective randomized crossover comparison of apical and outflow tract pacing. J Am Coll Cardiol 1999;33(2):311–6.

10. Tse HF, Yu C, Wong KK, et al. Functional abnormalities in patients with permanent right ventricular pacing: the effect of sites of electrical stimulation. J Am Coll Cardiol 2002;40(8):1451–8.

11. Occhetta E, Bortnik M, Magnani A, et al. Prevention of ventricular desynchronization by permanent para-hisian pacing after atrioventricular node ablation in chronic atrial fibrillation. J Am Coll Cardiol 2006; 47(10):1938–45.

12. Vassallo JA, Cassidy DM, Miller JM, et al. Left ventricular endocardial activation during right ventricular pacing: effect of underlying heart disease. J Am Coll Cardiol 1986;7(6):1228–33.

13. Eschalier R, Ploux S, Lumens J, et al. Detailed analysis of ventricular activation sequences during right ventricular apical pacing and left bundle branch block and the potential implications for cardiac resynchronization therapy. Heart Rhythm 2015;12(1): 137–43.

14. Badke FR, Boinay P, Covell JW. Effects of ventricular pacing on regional left ventricular performance in the dog. Am J Physiol 1980;238(6):H858–67.

15. Prinzen FW, Hunter WC, Wyman BT, et al. Mapping of regional myocardial strain and work during ventricular pacing: experimental study using magnetic resonance imaging tagging. J Am Coll Cardiol 1999;33(6):1735–42.

16. Owen CH, Esposito DJ, Davis JW, et al. The effects of ventricular pacing on left ventricular geometry, function, myocardial oxygen consumption, and efficiency of contraction in conscious dogs. Pacing Clin Electrophysiol 1998;21(7):1417–29.

17. Catanzariti D, Maines M, Cemin C, et al. Permanent direct his bundle pacing does not induce ventricular dyssynchrony unlike conventional right ventricular apical pacing. An intrapatient acute comparison study. J Interv Card Electrophysiol 2006;16(2):81–92.

18. Kronborg MB, Poulsen SH, Mortensen PT, et al. Left ventricular performance during para-His pacing in patients with high-grade atrioventricular block: an acute study. Europace 2012;14(6):841–6.

19. Catanzariti D, Maines M, Manica A, et al. Permanent His-bundle pacing maintains long-term ventricular synchrony and left ventricular performance, unlike conventional right ventricular apical pacing. Europace 2013;15(4):546–53.

20. Karpawich PP, Mital S. Comparative left ventricular function following atrial, septal, and apical single chamber heart pacing in the young. Pacing Clin Electrophysiol 1997;20(8 Pt 1):1983–8.

21. Cock CC, Meyer A, Kamp O, et al. Hemodynamic benefits of right ventricular outflow tract pacing: comparison with right ventricular apex pacing. Pacing Clin Electrophysiol 1998;21(3):536–41.

22. Mera F, DeLurgio DB, Patterson RE, et al. A comparison of ventricular function during high right ventricular septal and apical pacing after his-bundle ablation for refractory atrial fibrillation. Pacing Clin Electrophysiol 1999;22(8):1234–9.

23. Victor F, Mabo P, Mansour H, et al. A randomized comparison of permanent septal versus apical right ventricular pacing: short-term results. J Cardiovasc Electrophysiol 2006;17(3):238–42.

24. Leong DP, Mitchell A-M, Salna I, et al. Long-term mechanical consequences of permanent right ventricular pacing: effect of pacing site. J Cardiovasc Electrophysiol 2010;21(10):1120–6.

25. Zou C, Song J, Li H, et al. Right ventricular outflow tract septal pacing is superior to right ventricular apical pacing. J Am Heart Assoc 2015;4(4):e001777.

26. Padeletti L, Lieberman R, Schreuder J, et al. Acute effects of His bundle pacing versus left ventricular and right ventricular pacing on left ventricular function. Am J Cardiol 2007;100(10):1556–60.

His Bundle Pacing for Cardiac Resynchronization

Gaurav A. Upadhyay, MD, Roderick Tung, MD*

KEYWORDS

- Cardiac resynchronization therapy • His bundle pacing • Biventricular pacing
- Left bundle branch block

KEY POINTS

- His bundle pacing (HBP) successfully corrects QRS width by restoring physiologic ventricular activation in 75% to 90% of patients with typical bundle branch block.
- Short-term clinical data on the impact of HBP on clinical outcome, particularly echocardiographic improvement, appears promising.
- Current tools and technology to achieve HBP are still limited, and the ease of implant and clinical success may be improved by variable-shape sheath delivery systems and lead helix design.
- The mechanism for QRS correction remains unclear. Although longitudinal dissociation of the predestined fibers within the His bundle has been proposed, focal proximal block of the left bundle has been observed.

INTRODUCTION AND HISTORY OF PACING FOR RESYNCHRONIZATION

The introduction of cardiac resynchronization therapy (CRT) in the mid-1990s represented a paradigm shift for device-based electrical therapy in systolic heart failure.[1] The deleterious impact of right ventricular (RV) pacing had already been recognized,[2] and there was a growing awareness of the importance of minimizing RV pacing for patients with preserved normal ventricular activation and narrow QRS. In parallel, patients with dyssynchrony from left bundle branch block (LBBB),[3] were demonstrated to improve from biventricular pacing via synchronized RV and left ventricular (LV) coronary sinus pacing with QRS duration narrowing, improved mechanical synchrony, and augmented cardiac output.[4,5] Taken together, biventricular pacing eventually became the mainstay approach to CRT, with the goal of forcing paced synchronization for every beat, rather than merely minimizing dyssynchrony induced by RV pacing.

The concept of biventricular pacing was initially met with some skepticism with regard to physiologic activation. Biventricular pacing achieves CRT through fusion of two wavefronts from endocardial activation from the RV lead with a nonphysiologic LV epicardial-to-endocardial lateral wall activation from a tributary of the coronary sinus or a surgically placed LV lead. Early investigators paved the way for future randomized studies in CRT with coronary (CS) leads by demonstrating clinical feasibility of this approach in patients with severe heart failure, and validated improvements in quality of life from optimized pumping efficiency and LV energetics.[5–7] Interestingly, although there had been historical precedent to use His bundle pacing (HBP) to correct LBBB since the late 1970s,[8] the concept of engaging the His-Purkinje system directly with permanent HBP to restore physiologic electromechanical activation of the heart did not gain momentum during this period. This is notable in that biventricular pacing took hold as an approach despite the lack of specialized pacing systems or delivery tools for CS leads.

In the ensuing two decades, large randomized controlled trials (RCTs) led to approval of CRT-D systems as a treatment of choice for patients

The University of Chicago Medicine, Center for Arrhythmia Care, Heart and Vascular Center, 5841 South Maryland Avenue, Chicago, IL 60637, USA
* Corresponding author. Center for Arrhythmia Care, Heart and Vascular Center, The University of Chicago Medicine, 5841 South Maryland Avenue, MC 6080, Chicago, IL 60637.
E-mail address: rodericktung@uchicago.edu

Card Electrophysiol Clin 10 (2018) 511–517
https://doi.org/10.1016/j.ccep.2018.05.010

with symptomatic heart failure with severe systolic dysfunction and LBBB. Even with improvements in lead delivery systems, nonresponse rates remain high. Between 30% and 40% of patients do not exhibit demonstrable clinical, echocardiographic, or functional benefit from biventricular pacing.[9,10] It is in this context that permanent HBP has reemerged as a potential alternative to conventional CRT with an LV lead. In this review, we appraise the data supporting the role for HBP in resynchronization, discuss definitions of QRS correction and theories regarding mechanism, as well as outline opportunities for future investigation.

EARLY CLINICAL DATA

Five years after the first report of permanent His bundle pacing in patients with normal QRS by Deshmukh and colleagues,[11] Moriña-Vázquez and colleagues[12] were the first to describe use of permanent HBP in a CRT-eligible patient in a case report in 2005. A 62-year-old woman had presented with complete atrioventricular (AV) block and LBBB, and an electrophysiology (EP) study was performed during which it was

fortuitously noted that high-output pacing from the His recording electrode demonstrated a narrow-paced complex that appeared to exhibit normal activation. During subsequent device implantation, a biventricular pacemaker had been planned, but the CS could not be cannulated. The investigators then used a series of manually shaped stylets to navigate an active-fix lead to the His region, which was successful at correcting the patient's LBBB with nonselective HBP. The patient did well in follow-up with both clinical and echocardiographic improvement in 6-month follow-up.

Since this initial case report, several subsequent case reports[13–18] followed and 5 cohort studies (**Table 1**)[19–23] on the use of HBP in CRT-eligible patient populations were published in the literature. Barba-Pichardo and colleagues[19] were the first to report a case series of permanent HBP among CRT-eligible patients in whom the CS could not be cannulated. In contrast to more recent cohorts of patients, they used Tendril leads (St. Jude Medical, Sylmar, CA), which required manual revision of stylets to navigate to the His region. Using this technique, LBBB correction could

Table 1
Case series of permanent HBP in CRT-eligible patients with prior bundle branch block

Author, Year	n	Indication	His Bundle Lead	Implant Success, %	Primary Outcome
Barba-Pichardo et al,[19] 2013	16	CRT implant failure	Tendril 1488T, 1788 TC, 1888 TC	56	During mean follow-up of 31.3 ± 21.5 mo, NYHA Class improved III→II and LVEF improved from 29%→36% (P<.05)
Lustgarten et al,[19] 2015	29	Crossover study of HBP and CS lead	SelectSecure 3830	59	Patients demonstrated similar NYHA Class reduction (2.0→1.9, P<.001) and LVEF improvement from 26%→32% (P = .043)
Su et al,[21] 2016	16	CRT implant failure	SelectSecure 3830	100	Clinical outcomes not reported. HB tip-RV coil configuration demonstrated better capture thresholds and R-wave sensing than dedicated bipolar or unipolar
Ajijola et al,[22] 2017	21	Primary HBP	SelectSecure 3830	76	NYHA Class III→II (P<.001) and LVEF improved from 27% ± 10% to 41% ± 13% (P<.001)
Sharma et al,[23] 2018	106 (48 with BBB)	CRT implant failure and primary HBP	SelectSecure 3830	90	Among all patients, NYHA Class 2.8 ± 0.5→1.8 ± 0.6 (P = .0001) and LVEF improved from 30% ± 10% to 43% ± 13% (P = .0001)

Abbreviations: BBB, bundle branch block; CRT, cardiac resynchronization therapy; CS lead, coronary lead; HBP, His bundle pacing; LVEF, left ventricular ejection fraction; NYHA, New York Heart Association; RV, right ventricular.

be achieved in 13 of 16 patients during implant, of whom the lead could be fixed to provide permanent HBP in 9 patients. There was substantial QRS correction seen with permanent HBP, with the mean QRS reduction from 166 ± 8 ms to 97 ± 9 ms (P<.01; range 85–110 ms).

More recent cohorts have opted for near exclusive use of the fixed helix screw 3830 lead (Select-Secure; Medtronic Inc, Minneapolis, MN) and lead delivery sheaths, particularly the fixed-curve C315His sheath or the deflectable C304SelectSite sheath (Medtronic Inc). Analogous to early developments in transvenous approaches for CS lead positioning, the development of a first-generation delivery sheath for His region targeting has allowed for increased success of permanent HBP, although barriers remain, particularly in patients with dilated cardiomyopathy with markedly enlarged right atria.

Lustgarten and colleagues[20] were the first investigators to compare outcomes between HBP and traditional CS pacing with a prospective elegant crossover study design. Their protocol used a Y-adaptor in which the His and CS lead were connected and both placed into the LV port. This allowed for a crossover analysis of patients in which response during resynchronization with HBP versus LV pacing could be compared. Twenty-nine patients were studied (28 with LBBB, 1 atypical right bundle branch block [RBBB]), with QRS narrowing achieved acutely in 21 (72% of total). They used the deflectable C304 sheath for His lead placement and permanent HBP could not be placed in 12 patients. Failure of conventional CS LV lead placement occurred in 1 patient. Of the remaining 17 patients, only 12 completed the year-long follow-up period. By adjusting pacing output, they crossed over patients at 6 months. Significant improvements were noted with respect to quality of life, New York Heart Association (NYHA) functional class, and 6-minute hall walk test for both HBP and LV pacing compared with baseline. LV ejection fraction also significantly improved for both groups, but with no significant differences when compared with one another. The conclusion of the study was that resynchronization with HBP was comparable to standard biventricular pacing. These observations were tempered due to dropout in the study, and the inability to exclude the possibility that stimulation was present at both sites given use of the Y-adaptor.

The next case series to evaluate HBP in patients with CRT was reported by Su and colleagues.[21] In this single-center study, they had found that HBP could fully correct complete LBBB, but the focus was not clinical outcomes, but rather optimal pacing configuration. It had been noted previously that patients with HBP often required higher pacing outputs and also suffered from low R-waves. They explored how best to optimize HBP pacing configuration. They evaluated 25 CRT-eligible patients, of whom 16 eventually underwent permanent HB lead placement. In follow-up, they evaluated 2 configurations: "integrated" bipolar (HB tip-to-RV ring) and unipolar (HB tip-to-can) at 1 and 3 months after follow-up. At implant, they also evaluated a dedicated bipolar setting (HB tip-to-HB ring). An integrated HB tip-to-RV coil configuration was associated with lower capture thresholds and higher sensed R-wave at all time points.

The first to report on a series of primary HBP in CRT-eligible patients (in lieu of a traditional LV lead) were Ajijola and colleagues.[22] Among 21 patients (17 LBBB, 4 RBBB), permanent HBP was successfully placed in 16 patients (or 76%). Echocardiographic and clinical outcomes were favorable, with mean left ventricular ejection fraction (LVEF) improvement from 27% ± 10% to 41% ± 13% (P<.001) and mean NYHA functional class improving from III to II (P<.001). Nonselective capture was achieved in most patients, and QRS duration improved by approximately 30% (baseline 181 ± 23 ms to 129 ± 13 ms, P<.0001) (**Fig. 1**).

Most recently, Sharma and colleagues[23] reported results combined from 5 centers in the largest retrospective case series of CRT-eligible patients. They identified 2 distinct cohorts of patients: patients in whom HBP was being used as a bailout for unsuccessful traditional CS lead placement (Group 1, 33 patients), and patients in who HBP was being used as a primary strategy in patients who were CRT eligible either due to high expected pacing rate, known upgrade due to high pacing burden, or those with preexisting bundle branch block (BBB) (Group 2, 73 patients). Implant success was high, with permanent HBP achieved in 95 (90%) of 106 patients with a low degree of lead-associated complications (7 of 95 patients or 7.3%). During a mean follow-up period of 14 months, there was significant improvement in LVEF was noted across patients, from 30% ± 10% to 43% ± 13% (P=.0001), as well as NYHA class from 2.8 ± 0.5 to 1.8 ± 0.6 (P=.0001). Preexisting BBB was present in 48 patients (45% of total cohort), with most demonstrating LBBB at baseline (36 patients). Significant QRS narrowing was achieved in patients with both preexisting LBBB and non-LBBB. Importantly, the threshold for narrowing of BBB was 2.0 ± 1.2 V at 1 ms, and selective HBP with correction was achieved in 19 patients.

DEFINITIONS FOR QRS CORRECTION

Until recently, there were no established guidelines regarding definitions for assessing QRS

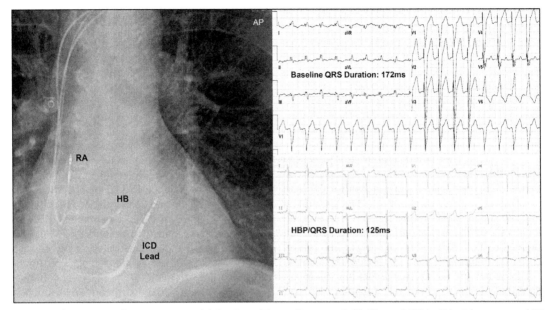

Fig. 1. Lead positions of CRT-D system with implantable cardioverter defibrillator (ICD) in RV midseptum and His lead placed at the annulus into the LV port. The right atrium (RA) is standard position in the RA appendage. QRS duration corrects from 172 ms with LBBB to 125 ms with nonselective His capture.

morphology during HBP. Indeed, prior work has adapted terminology from electrophysiology study (using phraseology such as para-His vs direct His capture), which has been imperfectly applied to patients undergoing permanent HBP. Recently, a multicenter collaborative work-group proposed a nomenclature to help unify terminology with respect to permanent HBP.[24] Broadly, the investigators identified 2 types of His bundle capture: selective and nonselective. Selective capture refers to scenarios in which the pacing stimulus captures only the His-Purkinje system (identified by isoelectric stimulus to QRS interval equivalent to the HV interval) and nonselective capture in which there is fusion between capture of the His-Purkinje system and adjacent ventricular myocardium (pseudodelta wave). Importantly, selective capture may be differentiated from nonselective capture by review of the His bundle electrogram on the pacing lead: the local ventricular electrogram is discrete and separated from the pacing stimulus in selective HBP, whereas it is fused with the pacing stimulus with nonselective capture.

Among patients with wide QRS undergoing HBP for resynchronization, additional terminology was proposed to categorize those with narrowing or QRS correction. Patients with QRS correction demonstrate a paced-QRS morphology that is narrower than the preexisting BBB. This may occur both for patients with selective and nonselective capture. Patients with nonselective HBP

may further demonstrate a third QRS morphology, that is, that of RV capture alone without apparent capture of the His-Purkinje system. Although selective HBP with correction is desirable, it is not achievable in all patients and may be present only over a narrow range of pacing outputs. Early data suggest selective and nonselective capture may be comparable clinically, as both have been associated with favorable outcomes, depending on the degree of ventricular fusion and time to His-Purkinje system engagement.[25,26]

POTENTIAL MECHANISMS OF QRS CORRECTION

The mechanism(s) of QRS correction in patients undergoing HBP for resynchronization remains unknown at present. Sherf and James[27] had proposed a concept of "sinoventricular conduction" in the late 1960s, in which impulses are predestined from the sinus node to specific areas in the ventricle. In an influential article from 1971, they presented their histologic observations (based on study of more than 400 human and 60 canine hearts) as well as observations from electron microscopy (from 1 human and 2 canine hearts).[28] They found that the human and canine His bundles were separated by fine collagen septa and proposed a concept of longitudinal separation of conduction in the His bundle. In the late 1970s, when Narula[8] was able to narrow the QRS of patients with preexisting LBBB at EP study with right-sided pacing, he hypothesized this was due to pacing just distal to proximal focal block on the right side. El-Sherif and colleagues[29] examined BBB patterns and normalization with distal HBP in 7 patients (4 with acute RBBB secondary to anterior wall myocardial infarction and 3 with chronic LBBB) and in 18 dogs (with ligation of anterior septal artery). Three of the patients demonstrated intra-His conduction delay and split His, and these patients could be narrowed with distal His pacing. Distal His pacing, or use of plunge electrode, further normalized BBB in 12 canines (or 67%). These observations supported the role for longitudinal dissociation of predestined fibers with evidence of intra-His delay as mechanism for QRS correction with right-sided pacing.

Subsequently, work by Lazzara and colleagues[30] called into question the notion of longitudinal dissociation. In an experiment with 5 excised portions of canine or rabbit hearts, they performed partial transections of the right or left bundle and found that activation distal to the lesion remained intact, with alterations only on the order of a few milliseconds. They proposed that functional transverse interconnections are numerous in the His bundle and the bundle branches, and that anatomic lesions did not lead to BBB. Bailey and colleagues[31] performed similar partial and complete transection studies in canines the following year. In these studies, they were able to demonstrate fast conduction from the isolated distal His bundle to the contralateral branch despite near complete transection. They found that functional interconnections allowed for propagation of a single, uniformly advancing wavefront, without longitudinal dissociation being present. Instead of an anatomic barrier, they proposed that functional dissociation may explain the findings, due to altered refractoriness or excitability, and does not require the presence of an anatomic obstacle.

Functionally, anisotropy of tissue and curvature may yield simultaneous depolarization and hyperpolarization of the cell membrane (the so-called "virtual electrode polarization effect" or VEP), and may result in both unidirectional block and reentry.[32–34] These situations are magnified around an isthmus, such as the bundle of His, leading to source-sink mismatch.[33,35] In this situation, functional block from VEP and source-to-sink mismatch may lead to isolated block of a bundle branch, and also overcome by pacing, as opposed to circumventing delay of a specific anatomic lesion.

Indeed, it may be that the etiology of LBBB or RBBB is heterogenous across patients. Certainly, for those with clearly identifiable intra-His disease, focal block of the isthmus might be overcome by HBP either distal to or capturing distal to a lesion. For patients without intra-His disease, however, it is possible that underlying cardiomyopathy might affect the transverse interconnections of the distal His and set up functional block of a bundle. This could be theoretically overcome by cathodal stimulation from the pacing lead at supraphysiologic outputs. Further study, particularly with respect to detailed left-sided recording, might better distinguish between intra-Hisian anatomic and infra-Hisian functional location of block.

FUTURE DIRECTIONS

Analogous to the early days of clinical investigation of biventricular pacing, there remain a number of questions with respect to use of HBP in CRT-eligible patients. Perhaps most critically, HBP must be compared directly with CRT with traditional CS or epicardial LV leads to assess clinical impact. The ongoing HIS-SYNC Pilot (NCT02700425) comparing HBP to conventional CRT with biventricular pacing is evaluating this question. Two other acute studies in patients with heart failure (HF) are also under way: the Electrical Resynchronization and Acute Hemodynamic Effects of Direct His Bundle Pacing Compared to Biventricular Pacing study (NCT03452462) will use noninvasive electrocardiographic imaging to compare and His Bundle Pacing in Bradycardia and Heart Failure (NCT03008291) will evaluate acute electrocardiographic metrics with HBP in patients undergoing CRT or dual-chamber implants. Other trials are exploring related questions in CRT-eligible patients, such as HOPE-HF (NCT02671903), which is evaluating use of HBP in patients with HF with long AV delay and without BBB, and the Comparison of His Bundle Pacing and Bi-Ventricular Pacing in Heart Failure With Atrial Fibrillation (NCT02805465). Although not pursuing HBP in patients with bundle branch disease, these and other trials will improve our understanding of HBP with respect to longer-term outcomes. Further study with large RCTs are also clearly needed to best elucidate appropriate patient selection and intraprocedural His lead targeting, as well as postimplant follow-up care and management.

With respect to patient selection, the use of HBP in patients with intraventricular conduction delay (IVCD) in particular remains uncertain. In contrast to biventricular pacing, in which final QRS width has only loosely been associated with outcome, degree of QRS correction is felt to mediate response from HBP. From first principles, this may not be achievable in patients with intact Purkinje activation and myocardial delay as a cause for IVCD. Intraprocedural lead targeting also needs to be clarified. Given that selective HBP with correction may not be achievable for all patients, to what extent is nonselective HBP with correction (or partial correction) still beneficial? Are relatively long pseudodelta waves before His-Purkinje engagement associated with similarly beneficial outcomes? What threshold should be accepted before abandoning an HBP strategy in favor of traditional CS targeting? Alternatively, could a more distal His-Purkinje target such as the proximal left bundle also be associated with benefit?

With regard to postimplant care, how should patients be followed and evaluated at device checks? What is an appropriate safety threshold for an HBP lead and when is it safe to reduce outputs? This is particularly notable, as a late rise in capture thresholds has been reported across case series. Furthermore, what is a reasonable time frame to wait for expected clinical benefit? Although early benefits have been noted in some patients, others have required extended periods of pacing for favorable ventricular remodeling over 6 to 12 months, similar to biventricular pacing.

The ability to reproducibly capture and preserve the intrinsic His-Purkinje activation in patients with narrow and wide QRS has reignited a new wave of enthusiasm for HBP. Preliminary reports suggest that more than 75% of cases of LBBB may be corrected by HBP. What remains unclear is the fundamental mechanism of how pacing proximal to a site of block can alleviate the bundle branch. Studies of high-density left septal mapping are ongoing at our institution. Improved implantation tools and prospective randomized trials are critically important to deliver on the promise of physiologic pacing in clinical practice.

REFERENCES

1. Cazeau S, Ritter P, Bakdach S, et al. Four chamber pacing in dilated cardiomyopathy. Pacing Clin Electrophysiol 1994;17(11 Pt 2):1974–9.
2. Rosenqvist M, Isaaz K, Botvinick EH, et al. Relative importance of activation sequence compared to atrioventricular synchrony in left ventricular function. Am J Cardiol 1991;67(2):148–56.
3. Grines CL, Bashore TM, Boudoulas H, et al. Functional abnormalities in isolated left bundle branch block. The effect of interventricular asynchrony. Circulation 1989;79(4):845–53.
4. Foster AH, Gold MR, McLaughlin JS. Acute hemodynamic effects of atrio-biventricular pacing in humans. Ann Thorac Surg 1995;59(2):294–300.
5. Cazeau S, Ritter P, Lazarus A, et al. Multisite pacing for end-stage heart failure: early experience. Pacing Clin Electrophysiol 1996;19(11 Pt 2):1748–57.
6. Leclercq C, Cazeau S, Le Breton H, et al. Acute hemodynamic effects of biventricular DDD pacing in patients with end-stage heart failure. J Am Coll Cardiol 1998;32(7):1825–31.
7. Kass DA, Chen CH, Curry C, et al. Improved left ventricular mechanics from acute VDD pacing in patients with dilated cardiomyopathy and ventricular conduction delay. Circulation 1999;99(12):1567–73.
8. Narula OS. Longitudinal dissociation in the His bundle. Bundle branch block due to asynchronous conduction within the His bundle in man. Circulation 1977;56(6):996–1006.
9. Mullens W, Grimm RA, Verga T, et al. Insights from a cardiac resynchronization optimization clinic as part of a heart failure disease management program. J Am Coll Cardiol 2009;53(9):765–73.
10. Brignole M, Auricchio A, Baron-Esquivias G, et al. 2013 ESC guidelines on cardiac pacing and cardiac resynchronization therapy: the Task Force on cardiac pacing and resynchronization therapy of the European Society of Cardiology (ESC). Developed in collaboration with the European Heart Rhythm Association (EHRA). Eur Heart J 2013;34(29):2281–329.
11. Deshmukh P, Casavant DA, Romanyshyn M, et al. Permanent, direct His-bundle pacing: a novel approach to cardiac pacing in patients with normal His-Purkinje activation. Circulation 2000;101(8):869–77.
12. Moriña-Vázquez P, Barba-Pichardo R, Venegas-Gamero J, et al. Cardiac resynchronization through selective His bundle pacing in a patient with the so-called InfraHis atrioventricular block. Pacing Clin Electrophysiol 2005;28(7):726–9.
13. Dabrowski P, Kleinrok A, Kozluk E, et al. Physiologic resynchronization therapy: a case of his bundle pacing reversing physiologic conduction in a patient with CHF and LBBB during 2 years of observation. J Cardiovasc Electrophysiol 2011;22(7):813–7.
14. Manovel A, Barba-Pichardo R, Tobaruela A. Electrical and mechanical cardiac resynchronisation by novel direct his-bundle pacing in a heart failure patient. Heart Lung Circ 2011;20(12):769–72.
15. Rehwinkel AE, Muller JG, Vanburen PC, et al. Ventricular resynchronization by implementation of direct his bundle pacing in a patient with congenital complete AV block and newly diagnosed cardiomyopathy. J Cardiovasc Electrophysiol 2011;22(7):818–21.
16. Wu G, Cai Y, Huang W, et al. Hisian pacing restores cardiac function. J Electrocardiol 2013;46(6):676–8.
17. Shan P, Su L, Chen X, et al. Direct His-bundle pacing improved left ventricular function and remodelling in a biventricular pacing nonresponder. Can J Cardiol 2015. https://doi.org/10.1016/j.cjca.2015.10.024.
18. Ajijola OA, Romero J, Vorobiof G, et al. Hyperresponse to cardiac resynchronization with permanent

His bundle pacing: is parahisian pacing sufficient? HeartRhythm Case Rep 2015;1(6):429–33.

19. Barba-Pichardo R, Manovel Sanchez A, Fernandez-Gomez JM, et al. Ventricular resynchronization therapy by direct His-bundle pacing using an internal cardioverter defibrillator. Europace 2013;15(1):83–8.

20. Lustgarten DL, Crespo EM, Arkhipova-Jenkins I, et al. His-bundle pacing versus biventricular pacing in cardiac resynchronization therapy patients: a crossover design comparison. Heart Rhythm 2015; 12(7):1548–57.

21. Su L, Xu L, Wu SJ, et al. Pacing and sensing optimization of permanent His-bundle pacing in cardiac resynchronization therapy/implantable cardioverter defibrillators patients: value of integrated bipolar configuration. Europace 2016;18(9):1399–405.

22. Ajijola OA, Upadhyay GA, Macias C, et al. Permanent His-bundle pacing for cardiac resynchronization therapy: initial feasibility study in lieu of left ventricular lead. Heart Rhythm 2017;14(9):1353–61.

23. Sharma PS, Dandamudi G, Herweg B, et al. Permanent His-bundle pacing as an alternative to biventricular pacing for cardiac resynchronization therapy: a multicenter experience. Heart Rhythm 2018;15(3):413–20.

24. Vijayaraman P, Dandamudi G, Zanon F, et al. Permanent His bundle pacing: recommendations from a multicenter His bundle pacing collaborative working group for standardization of definitions, implant measurements, and follow-up. Heart Rhythm 2018; 15(3):460–8.

25. Upadhyay GA, Tung R. Selective versus non-selective His bundle pacing for cardiac resynchronization therapy. J Electrocardiol 2017;50(2):191–4.

26. Zhang J, Guo J, Hou X, et al. Comparison of the effects of selective and non-selective His bundle pacing on cardiac electrical and mechanical synchrony. Europace 2017. https://doi.org/10.1093/europace/eux120.

27. Sherf L, James TN. A new electrocardiographic concept: synchronized sinoventricular conduction. Dis chest 1969;55(2):127–40.

28. James TN, Sherf L. Fine structure of the His bundle. Circulation 1971;44(1):9–28.

29. El-Sherif N, Amay YLF, Schonfield C, et al. Normalization of bundle branch block patterns by distal His bundle pacing. Clinical and experimental evidence of longitudinal dissociation in the pathologic His bundle. Circulation 1978; 57(3):473–83.

30. Lazzara R, Yeh BK, Samet P. Functional transverse interconnections within the His bundle and the bundle branches. Circ Res 1973;32(4): 509–15.

31. Bailey JC, Spear JF, Moore EN. Functional significance of transverse conducting pathways within the canine bundle of His. Am J Cardiol 1974;34(7):790–5.

32. Gray RA, Iyer A, Berenfeld O, et al. Interdependence of virtual electrode polarization and conduction velocity during premature stimulation. J Electrocardiol 2006;39(4 Suppl):S13–8.

33. Laurita KR, Rosenbaum DS. Interdependence of modulated dispersion and tissue structure in the mechanism of unidirectional block. Circ Res 2000; 87(10):922–8.

34. Sepulveda NG, Roth BJ, Wikswo JP Jr. Current injection into a two-dimensional anisotropic bidomain. Biophys J 1989;55(5):987–99.

35. Smaill BH, Zhao J, Trew ML. Three-dimensional impulse propagation in myocardium: arrhythmogenic mechanisms at the tissue level. Circ Res 2013; 112(5):834–48.

Pacing Treatment of Atrial Fibrillation Patients with Heart Failure

His Bundle Pacing Combined with Atrioventricular Node Ablation

Weijian Huang, MD, FHRS[a,b,*], Lan Su, MD[a,b],
Shengjie Wu, MD[a,b]

KEYWORDS

- Atrial fibrillation • Heart failure • His bundle pacing • Atrioventricular node ablation

KEY POINTS

- His bundle pacing (HBP) can preserve/restore ventricular synchrony. HBP combined with atrioventricular node (AVN) ablation is demonstrated feasible, effective, and suitable for atrial fibrillation (AF) patients with heart failure (HF) who suffer from insufficient or unbearable medication therapy or failed AF catheter ablation, especially in those with other arrhythmias that need pacemaker therapy.
- In patients who undergo AVN ablation, pacing in the distal His bundle or bundle branch allows adequate space for AVN ablation.
- Ablate from atrial side to keep sufficient safety distance to pacing site, preserving the pacing function of HBP lead.
- Prospective, randomized controlled studies are needed to compare AVN ablation and HBP with medical therapy and AF ablation.

INTRODUCTION

The estimated number of individuals with atrial fibrillation (AF) in 2010 was 33.5 million globally and increases by 5 million each year.[1] The main risk of AF includes thromboembolism, heart failure (HF), and dementia.[2–5] Previous investigations have demonstrated that HF and AF coexist in approximately 13% to 27% HF patients.[6] Patients with AF and HF have a higher risk of thromboembolic events and a higher mortality compared with those with only AF or HF.[7,8] Established treatment of AF includes upstream therapy[9] of concomitant conditions, anticoagulation, and rate/rhythm management. Nowadays the main methods to achieve rate/rhythm control include pharmacologic therapy, AF ablation, and atrioventricular node (AVN) ablation in combination with pacing therapy. How to control heart rate/rhythm individually, however, is the most important and debatable key point.[10] Therefore, this article reviews the methods for rate/rhythm control and focuses on the clinical application of His bundle pacing (HBP) plus AVN ablation in AF patients with HF as well as relevant skills associated with HBP lead implantation and AVN ablation.

CURRENT STATE OF RATE/RHYTHM CONTROL

Currently, 3 strategies to control heart rate and rhythm in AF patients are pharmacotherapy,

Competing Interests Statement: All have no conflicts.
a Department of Cardiology, The First Affiliated Hospital of Wenzhou Medical University, Nanbaixiang, Wenzhou 325000, China; b Key Lab of Cardiovascular Disease of Wenzhou, Nanbaixiang, Wenzhou 325000, China
* Corresponding author. Department of Cardiology, The First Affiliated Hospital of Wenzhou Medical University, Nanbaixiang, Wenzhou 325000, China.
E-mail address: weijianhuang69@126.com

Card Electrophysiol Clin 10 (2018) 519–535
https://doi.org/10.1016/j.ccep.2018.05.016
1877-9182/18/© 2018 Elsevier Inc. All rights reserved.

catheter ablation of AF, and pacemaker implantation post–AVN ablation. Feasibility and effectiveness of these 3 therapies have been clinically demonstrated.

Pharmacotherapy

Pharmacotherapy as the initial strategy for rate/rhythm control has been practiced for quite a while, but disadvantages of pharmacotherapy of AF have been universally acknowledged. The successful rate of restoring and maintaining sinus rhythm is low. The subgroup analysis of AFFIRM trial showed that recurrence rate of AF in patients with abnormal ejection fraction (EF) was fairly high and up to 84%.[11] Some antiarrhythmic drugs (ADDs) used for AF rhythm control, including dronedarone, may make HF worse.[12,13] Meta-analyses indicate that except for β-blockers, most ADDs for heart rate control, including calcium channel blockers and digoxin, increase mortality.[14,15] Results from the Rate Control Efficacy in Permanent Atrial Fibrillation: a Comparison between Lenient versus Strict Rate Control II (RACE II) study indicated that in patients with permanent atrial fibrillation, lenient rate control with resting heart rate <110 beats per minute(bpm) is as effective as strict rate control with resting heart rate <80 bpm and heart rate during moderate exercise <110 bpm; the frequencies of the primary outcome were similar in the 2 groups.[16] One reason likely was the adverse effects of drugs for rate control, and another reason was the low quality of rate control by drugs. Low mean ventricular rate does not stand for regular rhythm whereas irregular rhythm during AF under rate control is another important factor causing cardiac dysfunction.

Catheter Ablation of Atrial Fibrillation

Previous research findings[17–20] with small sample size were similar in outcome to the results of the recently published Catheter Ablation vs. Standard Conventional Treatment in Patients With LV Dysfunction and AF (CASTLE-AF) trial. Catheter ablation of AF in patients with reduced EF is associated with improved all-cause mortality and fewer admissions for worsening HF compared with conventional treatment.[21] Successful rate of cardioversion to maintain sinus rhythm are impacted by multiple factors, such as the mechanism of AF, underlying cardiac disease, size and fibrosis of left atrium (LA), and duration of AF.[21–23] A meta-analysis[24] evaluating the long-term outcome of 6167 patients who underwent a single radiofrequency ablation procedure for AF revealed that only 54.1% of paroxysmal AF patients and 41.8% of nonparoxysmal AF patients maintained sinus rhythm. Generally speaking, AF ablation in patients with HF is challenging due to issues, including lack of effective methods to monitor heart rhythm after ablation, high recurrence rate of AF in patients with large LA and long duration of AF, high cost of repeated catheter ablation to maintain sinus rhythm, and procedure-related complications.

Atrioventricular Node Ablation

Experience with AVN ablation and pacing for AF patients who are nonresponders or intolerant to intensive rate and rhythm control therapy includes more than 20 years of therapy.[25] A meta-analysis from Wood and colleagues[25] using data from 10 studies, including 41% to 54% of patients with paroxysmal AF, showed that radiofrequency ablation of the AVN and permanent pacing could improve exercise duration/ventricular function/quality of life and symptoms compared with medical therapy alone. Although AVN ablation improves symptoms, long-term right ventricular (RV) apical pacing produces left ventricular (LV) dyssynchrony and hemodynamic impairment.[26] For some patients, RV apical pacing can lead to pacing-induced cardiomyopathy.[27] The PAVE study (Left ventricular-based cardiac stimulation post AV nodal ablation evaluation) and AVAIL CLS/CRT trial (AV-node Ablation With CLS and CRT Pacing Therapies for the Treatment of AF)[28–30] and meta-analysis[31] demonstrated superior outcomes with biventricular pacing (BVP) for preserving cardiac function compared to RV pacing. The guidelines for cardiac resynchronization therapy (CRT) from the European Society of Cardiology (ESC) in 2013[32] and American Heart Association (AHA)/American College of Cardiology (ACC)/Heart Rhythm Society (HRS) in 2014[33] both recommend that BVP is considered for HF patients unresponsive or intolerant to intensive rate and rhythm control therapy (Class IIa, level of evidence: B). For patients whose intrinsic QRS duration is less than 130 ms after AVN ablation, not enough evidence supports BVP to maintain synchronization of ventricular contraction, and BVP may even induce desynchrony.[34,35] One limitation to BVP is this pacing is not truly physiologic especially in patients with a narrow QRS complex. Recent investigations[36] have found that HBP can provide physiologic ventricular activation and hence avoids ventricular dyssynchrony and preserves ventricular function in AF patients with normal His-Purkinje conduction system.

In 2000, Deshmukh and colleagues[37] first reported successful AVN ablation and permanent direct HBP in AF patients. Since then, there have been multiple studies with small sample sizes that show similar results probing that AVN ablation and permanent HBP is clinically feasible, safe, and effective. A recent study (n = 42) by Huang and colleagues[38] demonstrated that during a median follow-up of 20 months, permanent HBP in conjunction with AVN ablation leads to significantly improved echocardiographic measurements and New York Heart Association (NYHA) classification and reduced diuretic use for HF. This was found true regardless of whether patients with a narrow QRS who had either HF with reduced EF or HF with preserved EF. The successful rate of HBP was 96.2% in the subgroup with LVEF less than or equal to 40%; the percentage increase in LVEF (the ratio of LVEF at 1-year HBP over the baseline value) was 82.8% ± 43.3% in HF with reduced EF patients. Compared with the baseline, HBP thresholds and sensed R wave did not significantly change during follow-up and the percentage of HBP remained at 99% during follow-up. This study implied HBP combined with AVN ablation continues to produce benefits of LV reverse remodeling and cardiac function improvement in long-standing AF patients even with relatively good rate control at a mean heart rate 83.9 bpm ± 14.1 bpm using optimal pharmacotherapy. Vijayaraman and colleagues[39] reported HBP was successful in 40 of 42 patients (95%); LVEF increased significantly; and HBP was feasible, safe, and effective during the mean follow-up time of 19 months. Thus, the primary choice of pacing mode after AVN ablation should be HBP, because HBP has a distinct advantage over BVP and RV pacing (RVP) in preserving ventricular systolic synchrony for patients with a normal QRS duration. Additionally, HBP can correct complete left bundle branch block (CLBBB), which benefits patients with left bundle branch block (LBBB). At present, HBP is becoming more popularized in clinical practice with technology improvement, including implantation in the distal part of His bundle and deeper fixation technology that solves problems of high-threshold, low-sensing amplitude, and long-term safety. HBP seems more feasible and better than BVP, which needs more research clinical data to confirm.

The current experience in AVN ablation combined with HBP for AF patients is mostly from single-center studies, so large, prospective, randomized controlled trials need to be designed to provide strong evidence to evaluate efficacy and safety of AVN ablation with HBP compared with drug therapy, AVN ablation and BVP, and catheter ablation of AF.

Complete Atrioventricular (AV) block by AVN ablation is mainly recommended for patients with long-standing persistent AF when pharmacologic therapy is inadequate and rhythm control is not achievable. AVN ablation is not recommended for patients with AF caused by reversible underlying diseases, such as hyperthyroidism, acute valvular disease, acute myocardial infarction, and electrolyte and internal environment disturbance. The recommendation of AVN ablation in guidelines is shown in **Table 1**.

Current recommendations from guidelines are unclear. In particular, AV node ablation may be considered when the rate cannot be controlled and tachycardia-mediated cardiomyopathy is suspected.

Table 1
American Heart Association/American College of Cardiology/Heart Rhythm Society and European Society of Cardiology guidelines for the use of atrioventricular node ablation for ventricular rate control in atrial fibrillation

Atrioventricular node ablation for ventricular rate control		
2014 AHA/ACC/HRS guideline for the management of patients with atrial fibrillation[32]	AV node ablation with permanent ventricular pacing is reasonable to control heart rate when pharmacologic therapy is inadequate and rhythm control is not achievable.	IIa, B
2016 ESC guidelines for the management of atrial fibrillation developed in collaboration with European Association for Cardio-Thoracic Surgery[40]	AV node ablation should be considered to control heart rate in patients unresponsive or intolerant to intensive rate and rhythm control therapy, accepting that these patients will become pacemaker dependent.	IIa, B
Atrioventricular node ablation for ventricular rate control in patients with heart failure and atrial fibrillation		
2014 AHA/ACC/HRS guideline for the management of patients with atrial fibrillation[33]	It is reasonable to perform AV node ablation with ventricular pacing to control heart rate when pharmacologic therapy is insufficient or not tolerated.	IIa, B
	AV node ablation may be considered when the rate cannot be controlled and tachycardia-mediated cardiomyopathy is suspected.	IIb, C

In conclusion, the most optimal therapy for AF is to restore sinus rhythm. Successful cardioversion and sinus rhythm maintenance, however, are infrequently achieved. AVN ablation in conjunction with pacing therapy has become one approach to achieve strict management of ventricular rate/rhythm control for a lifetime especially when using HBP, which produces physiologic ventricular activation (**Table 2**).

AVN ablation combined with HBP should be considered for patients having following factors (**Box 1**).

PROCEDURE AND METHODS OF HIS BUNDLE PACING AND ATRIOVENTRICULAR NODE ABLATION
Implant Procedures

The 2014 AHA/ACC/HRS guideline[33] for the management of patients with AF recommends that pacemaker implantation may be performed 4 weeks to 6 weeks before AVN ablation to ensure proper pacemaker function and avoid possible catastrophic device malfunction, such as lead dislodgment. The authors recommend performing AVN ablation after HBP at the same time (**Fig. 1**) with the following considerations. First, for AF patients with HF who receive HBP combined with AVN ablation, successful HBP is the prerequisite for AVN ablation. Second, the His pacing lead can be used as a landmark to guide radiofrequency catheter for AVN ablation to avoid damage to the HIS pacing site and distal conduction to ventricles. Third, it is easy to monitor and detect damage to the pacing lead real time. In the authors' experience, lead dislodgement rarely occurs during AVN ablation, but in case the HBP threshold increases, the His lead can be repositioned. The outline for the procedure is shown in **Figs. 2** and **3**.

The reason why both procedures are done at 1 time is as follows: (1) the authors believe it is safe to do because lead dislodgment happens rarely in the previous research and in the authors' center, especially for patients with backup pacing; (2) in case threshold of HBP increases to an inacceptable degree during AVN ablation, it is easy to reposition pacing lead; (3) HBP threshold has been getting low and stable as technology develops; and (4) radiofrequency catheter can be used for HIS potential mapping to help HBP lead implantation in certain conditions. The procedure is as follows (see **Fig. 2**).

His Bundle Pacing Lead Implantation

Steps of His bundle pacing lead implantation
Choice of implantation HBP lead and device is as follows. The delivery sheath (model C304 or C315, Medtronic, Minneapolis, Minnesota) and the Select-Secure lead (model 3830, Medtronic, Minneapolis, Minnesota) are preferentially used for HBP reported by in almost all studies published since 2004. To choose the device, the following instructions should be considered. HBP lead is generally not connected

Table 2
Comparison of 3 main clinical therapies to treat atrial fibrillation patients with heart failure

	Antiarrhythmic Drugs	Catheter Ablation	Atrioventricular Node Ablation and Pacing
Restoration of sinus rhythm	Less effective	Effective depending on the basic cause	Loss of atrial rhythm
Ventricular rate/rhythm control	Less effective	Effective depending on the basic cause	Almost 100%
Impact on prognosis	Increased risk of worsening HF and mortality especially in patients with reduced LVEF except for β-blocker	Improved	Improved
Inappropriate shocks by AF in patients with ICD	Probable	Reduced but possible	Never
Intraventricular block including CLBBB	Not effective	Not effective	HBP or CRT could achieve resynchronization
Impact in ventricular synchronous contraction	No	No	Yes, depending on different ventricular pacing mode
Disadvantage	Side effects	High recurrent rate of AF	Need continuous pacing

<table>
<tbody>
<tr><td>

Box 1
Factors preferred for His bundle pacing combined with atrioventricular node ablation therapy

Patients who still have severe symptoms when pharmacologic therapy is inadequate and rhythm control is not achievable

Patients intolerant to side effects of the drug

Elderly patients or HF patients who refuse AF ablation

Patients with peculiar anatomic structure not suitable for catheter ablation: anomaly or occlusion of vena cava; after filter placement; after percutaneous amplatzer device closure of atrial septal defect

Contraindication to AF catheter ablation: left atrial appendage thrombus, contraindication to anticoagulant drugs

Patients with failed catheter ablation

Severe atrial disease: very large atrium; diffuse atrial fibrosis

Patients with inappropriate shocks by AF

Patients who have indication for device implantation

</td></tr>
</tbody>
</table>

to the IS-1 (an International Connector Standard, ISO 5841-3) port of implantable cardioverter defibrillator (ICD) due to the reliability of the R wave amplitude from the HBP lead. Choice of device type is determined by whether additional ventricular backup pacing, including BVP or RVP, is needed and whether the atrial lead is required for

implantation. The recommendations from the international HBP collaborative working group published in 2017 suggest that long-term pacing threshold was stable in recent studies.[41]

Special skills of HBP implantation

1. The dual-lead method is a technique using 2 sets of lead and delivery systems that can be applied for alternately mapping and locating optimal HIS pacing site to obtain a lower His capture threshold, to make it easy to fix the lead, and to increase the success rate of HBP lead implantation in less time.
2. Place the His lead in the distal portion of the His bundle to acquire lower and stable His capture thresholds and higher R-wave amplitude.
3. CLBBB correction by HBP has been reported by many groups[42–46] but the acute and long-term LBBB correction threshold is relatively high, at approximately 4 V/0.75 ms.[43] This problem could be solved by placing the pacing lead at a site distal to conduction delay.[47]

How to Ablate Atrioventricular Node to Achieve Complete Atrioventricular Block Ventricular

Many previous researchers demonstrated that ablation of the AVN is used to obtain complete AV block; however, only the AVN and a portion of the His bundle proximal to the pacing site no more than 8 mm can be used for ablation in AF patients with HBP. It is possible that use of 4-mm tip or open-irrigated ablation catheters could achieve deeper and wider lesions, resulting in successful

A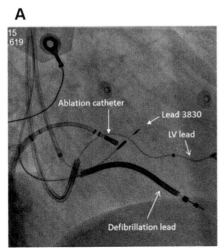

B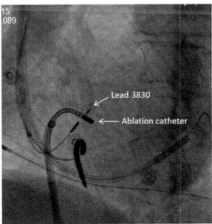

Fig. 1. Right (*A*) and left (*B*) anterior oblique fluoroscopic projections showing location of HBP lead and ablation catheter. (*From* Huang W, Su L, Wu S, et al. Benefits of permanent his bundle pacing combined with atrioventricular node ablation in atrial fibrillation patients with heart failure with both preserved and reduced left ventricular ejection fraction. J Am Heart Assoc 2017;6:e005309; with permission.)

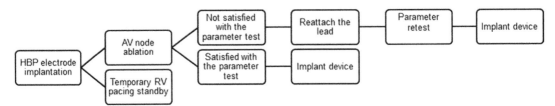

Fig. 2. Operative procedures.

AVN ablation while maintaining the catheter tip at or below the ring electrode of the HBP lead38,39 (ablation site seen in **Fig. 4**). Kulkarni and colleagues[48] reported 11 cases of AVN ablations followed by HBP at high output (10 mA at 2 ms) that initially achieved right bundle branch capture. The catheter was withdrawn until a narrow QRS morphology and radiofrequency (RF) energy was applied at the site of HBP capture until AV block was observed. The authors use an 8.5F-long sheath (SR0 or SL1, St. Jude Medical, St. Paul, Minnesota) or a deflectable sheath (Agilis, Abbott Electrophysiology, Menlo Park, California) to acquire better catheter tissue contact force, which is crucial for successful AVN ablation and durable AV block or if the right atrium is severely enlarged.[38]

The method the authors recommended to ablate the AV node is from the atrial side. The specific diagram is shown in **Fig. 4**.

The sign of effective ablation is the emerging of a transient rapid ventricular response; then the ventricular rate gradually slows down to a regular rate. Criteria of successful AVN ablation are as follows:[38]

1. Complete AV block is present.
2. No changes in HBP threshold and His ventricular conduction are seen.
3. The same morphology of the HBP QRS before and after AVN ablation.
4. Isoprenaline infusion (at 20–40 µg/min) over 10 minutes ensures no recurrence of AV conduction.
5. Occurrence of the escape rhythm. If the heart rate greater than 70 bpm, ablation should be reperformed until complete AV block is achieved.

Whether to Implant the Atrial Lead and How to Program Device After Procedure

Atrial lead should be reserved for patients with paroxysmal AF, and it is also considered for patients who may have chance to restore sinus rhythm or need atrioventricular sequence to maintain cardiac function and for some patients who have already implanted atrial lead before or intend to reserve atrial lead.

For programming the device appropriately after implantation, principles include

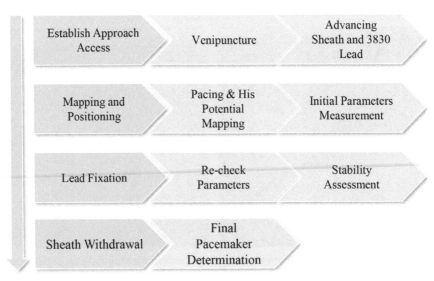

Fig. 3. Flow chart of standard implantation procedure: multiple parameters measurement to confirm the stability of the pacing parameters.

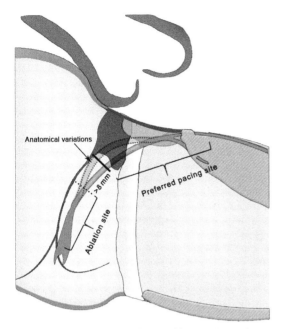

Fig. 4. Relative position of AVN ablation site and pacing site.

1. Setting of the base rate: the base rate of the HBP after AV node ablation should be based on baseline cardiac function, preoperative baseline heart rate, and the possibility of ventricular arrhythmias after implantation.
2. It is not recommended to set the immediate basic pacing rate below 80 bpm. It is reported there is a difference in the rate of sudden death when setting the rate less than 60 bpm comparing to decrease the rate step by step from 90 bpm ($P = .007$).[49]
3. Turning on the RV back-up pacing or not should be based on whether HBP pacing alone ensures patient safety.
4. Device with defibrillation feature: if the HBP lead is inserted into right atrial (RA) port and the device has defibrillation features, the authors do not use the dual-chamber ventricular tachycardia/ventricular fibrillation (VT/VF) discrimination algorithms. It may cause ventricular thrombosis/ventricular fibrillation to be undetected.
5. Because there are no specific devices for HBP, the programmable range of the device should be understood before the procedure and selecting the appropriate device.

CASE EXAMPLES
Patient 1

A 68-year-old woman experienced repetitive HF for more than 15 years. ECG showed AF (**Fig. 5**A) and echocardiogram revealed LVEF of 33%, LV end-diastolic diameter (LVEDd) of 76 mm, and LA of 67 mm. She was diagnosed with dilated cardiomyopathy, CLBBB, AF, and NYHA III. The authors decided to perform AVN ablation and pacemaker implantation in April 2016.

The RV lead was placed in the apex of RV. His capture threshold was 0.5 V/0.5 ms, and LBBB correction threshold was 2 V/0.5 ms, with sensing amplitude of 3.3 mV and impedance of 450 Ω (**Fig. 5**C, D). Local myocardial capture threshold was 3.25 V/0.5 ms. Complete AV block (**Fig. 5**B) was achieved using AVN ablation without affecting HBP parameters. Finally, a cardiac resynchronisation therapy-pacemaker(CRT-P, model C2TR01, Medtronic) was implanted with his lead connected to atrial port, RV lead in the septum of the RV connected to the RV port, and CS lead in lateral branch connected to LV port (model C2TR01, Medtronic). HBP with LBBB correction had narrower paced QRS duration compared to that of RVP and BVP (**Fig. 5**D–F). After 1-year follow-up, echocardiographic measurements were improved with an LVEF of 40%, LVEDd of 72 mm, and LA of 62 mm.

Take-home message:

1. His bundle was captured by a low pacing threshold, and LBBB corrected by a higher pacing output.

Patient 2

A 62-year-old woman with HF and repetitive AF despite optimal drug therapy underwent radiofrequency AF ablation in 2008, 2010, and 2012. Recently, an echocardiogram revealed an EF of 32% and LVEDd of 53 mm. She was diagnosed as having a dilated cardiomyopathy, AF, and NYHA class IV HF. AVN ablation and pacemaker implantation were performed for her as the treatment strategy in August 2012 (**Fig. 6**A–C).

After 5-year follow-up, heart function was improved to NYHA II and stable. Echocardiogram showed an EF of 44% and LVEDd of 48 mm and the heart-thoracic ratio improved (**Fig. 6**D, E). Pacing parameters remained stable.

Take-home messages:

1. Drug refractory and failed radiofrequency AF ablation
2. HBP and AVN ablation improved this patient's clinic symptoms and echo parameters in a long-term follow-up while the long-term pacing parameters of HBP maintained stability.

Patient 3

A 46-year-old man experienced symptomatic congestive HF (CHF) from dilated cardiomyopathy and chronic AF (**Fig. 7**A). In March 2009, he

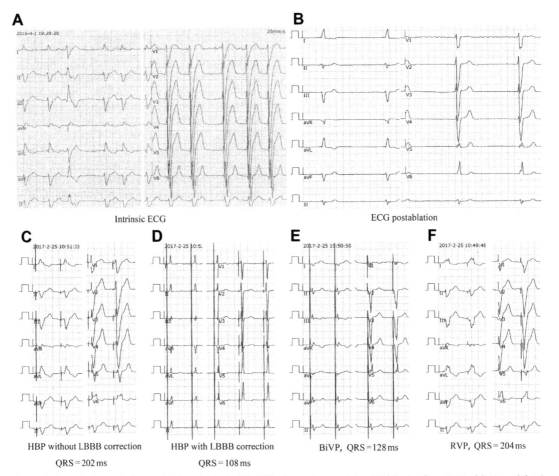

Fig. 5. (*A*) Intrinsic ECG showed AF and LBBB; (*B*) ECG showed complete AV block after AVN ablation; (*C*) His captured and (*D*) LBBB corrected by HBP; (*E*) BVP; and (*F*) RV pacing.

underwent AVN ablation and implantation of a CRT defibrillator. After AVN ablation, the electrocardiogram showed a ventricular escape rhythm with LBBB-like QRS morphology (**Fig. 7**B). Over a 4-year follow-up, the patient responded poorly to CRT (**Fig. 7**C,D) and underwent multiple hospitalizations for HF. Then, he was referred for upgrading to HBP in July 2013 with LVEF of 26% and LVEDd of 66 mm.

An additional pacing lead was placed at the His bundle region (**Fig. 7**F). HBP was achieved during pace mapping. The original right atrial lead was capped and abandoned. His lead was connected to atrial port, RV lead was placed in the RV apex connected to the RV port, and CS lead was placed in lateral branch connected to LV port (Cardiac Resynchronization Therapy Defibrillator [CRT-D], Model 3231–40, St. Jude Medical). After 2 years of follow-up, improvement in clinical outcomes was observed, including EF improved to 44%,

LVEDd to 55 mm and the heart-thoracic ratio decreased (**Fig. 7**G,H).

Take-home messages:

1. HPB improved cardiac function in CRT nonresponse patient.
2. HBP can rectify CLBBB by pace mapping in absence of His potential (**Fig. 7**D, E).

Patient 4

A 64-year-old woman presented with HF, diagnosed as AF and dilated cardiomyopathy. Her EF was 30% and underwent ICD implantation in Jan 2013. Since then, she still suffered from dyspnea and HF and had several inappropriate shocks due to AF with aberrant ventricular conduction. She was referred for upgrading to CRT-D and AVN ablation in September 2017.

At implantation, CS pacing lead was placed in anterior-lateral branch. During the procedure,

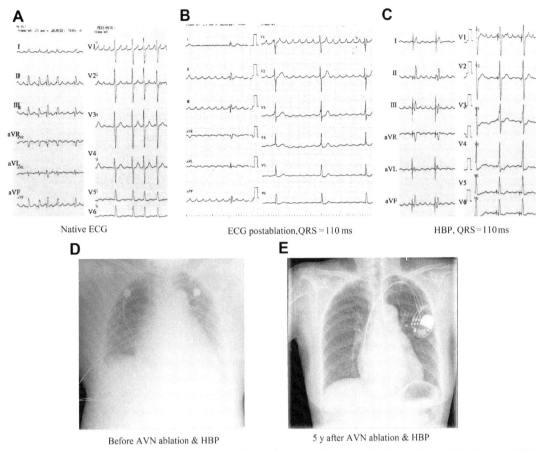

Fig. 6. (A) Native ECG showed AF; (B) ECG showed complete AV block after AVN ablation; (C) LBBB corrected by HBP; (D) radiograph of chest before HBP and (E) 5 years after HBP.

transient LBBB could not be corrected by HBP (**Fig. 8**A, B), so the authors placed the lead at left bundle branch (LBB) area with a threshold of 0.5 V/0.5 ms and paced QRS of RBBB pattern with 112 ms (see **Fig. 8**C, D). LBB lead was connected to atrial port, RV lead was placed in the septum of RV connected to RV port and CS lead was placed in anterior-lateral branch connected to LV port (CRT-D, D394TRG, Medtronic). The duration of BVP and RVP were 146 ms and 152 ms (**Fig. 8**E, F). Four months after LBB pacing only, her cardiac function improved from NYHA III to NYHA II and no inappropriate shocks occurred.

Take-home messages:

1. Patient with ICD who got inappropriate shocks due to AF can upgrade to HBP combined with AVN ablation.
2. Cardiac function improved

Patient 5

A 46-year-old man with symptomatic HF and refractory AF despite optimal drug control.

Echocardiography showed LVEF of 25%, LVEDd of 63 mm and LA of 48 mm. He was diagnosed with a dilated cardiomyopathy, AF with rapid ventricular rate, NYHA IV symptoms, and thus underwent HBP + AVN ablation in February 2018.

During the implantation procedure, the pacing lead was first placed in the His bundle region with a pacing output over 3 V/0.5 ms for selective HBP (**Fig. 9**A). Then, the pacing lead was moved distally to the LBB area where LBB area pacing was achieved at 0.5 V/0.5 ms (see **Fig. 9**B, C). AVN ablation was performed to achieve complete AV block with accelerating junctional rhythm during ablation (see **Fig. 9**D, E). LBB area pacing lead was connected to the atrial port of the CRT-D device (D384TRG, Medtronic).

Take-home messages:

1. Typical AVN ablation phenomenon with accelerating junctional rhythm during ablation (see **Fig. 9**D, E)

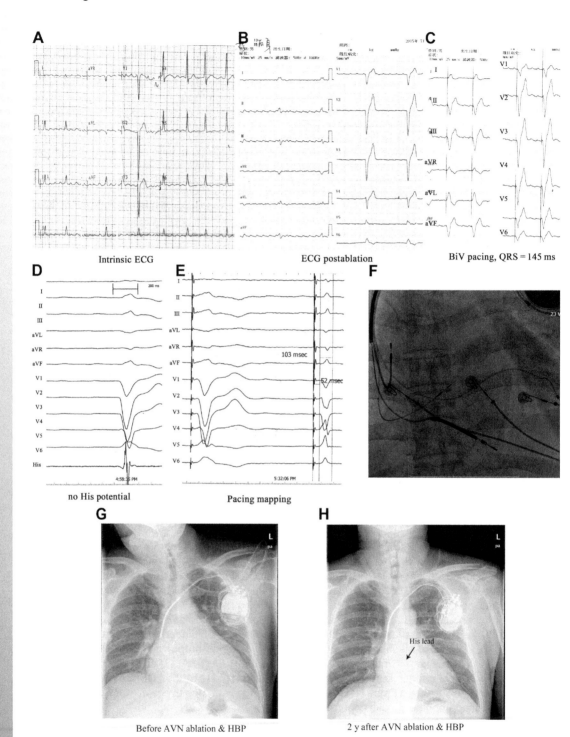

Fig. 7. (*A*) Native ECG showed AF; (*B*) ECG showed complete AV block after AVN ablation; (*C*) BVP before upgrading to HBP; (*D*) no His potential was observed in His electrogram; (*E*) LBBB was corrected using pace mapping; (*F*) fluoroscopic imaging of HBP and (*E*) radiograph before HBP and (*H*) 2 years after HBP.

2. LBB area pacing with low pacing threshold for LBBB correction (see **Fig. 9**C)
3. Dual-leads (HBP and LBB area pacing [see **Fig. 9**F, G])

Patient 6

A 78-year-old man had persistent AF and HF for 4 years. The ECG showed AF with a rapid ventricular rate and CLBBB (**Fig. 10**A). The

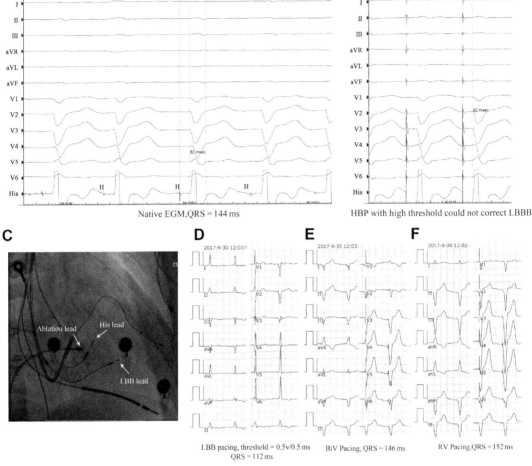

Fig. 8. (*A*) Native ECG showed AF; (*B*) high threshold cannot correct LBBB; (*C*) his lead and LBB area lead; (*D*) LBB area pacing with a threshold of 0.5 V/0.5 ms to correct LBBB; and (*E*) BVP and (*F*) RV pacing. EGM, electrogram.

echocardiogram showed an EF of 30%, LVEDd of 66 mm, and LA of 57 mm. He was diagnosed with cardiomyopathy and persistent AF and NYHA III and underwent AVN ablation. At the first pacing site, there was no LBBB correction at threshold of 3 V/0.5 ms. The second lead was placed in a nearby area with the LBBB correction threshold of 0.5 V/0.5 ms (**Fig. 10** E). The procedure caused transient infra-Hisian complete block (**Fig. 10**B). AVN ablation (**Fig. 10**F) was performed to achieve complete AV block along with the reduction of ventricular rate and disappearance of His potential (**Fig. 10**C, D). The His lead was connected to the atrial port, RV lead was placed in the RV apex connected to RV port, and CS lead was placed in anterior-lateral branch connected to LV port (CRT-D, D394TRG, Medtronic). Five months after HBP, his cardiac function improved from NYHA III to NYHA II with LVEF of 42%, LVEDd of 62 mm, and LA of 51 mm.

Take-home messages:

1. Dual lead method can be used to find ideal pacing site (**Fig. 10**E).
2. Transient infra-Hisian complete block caused by lead implantation (see **Fig. 10**B).
3. Reduction of rate and ultimate disappearance of His potential indicates successful AVN ablation that blocked the conduction from atrial to His bundle (see **Fig. 10**C, D).

Patient 7

A 74-year-old man had a history of persistent AF (**Fig. 11**A) for 6 years and HF for 4 years. Echocardiogram showed an EF of 35%. He was diagnosed with a dilated cardiomyopathy, persistent AF, and NYHA III HF. Rate control was judged adequate. The authors performed CRT-D implantation and AVN ablation in January 2016.

After HBP implantation, complete AV block could not be achieved using irrigated ablation

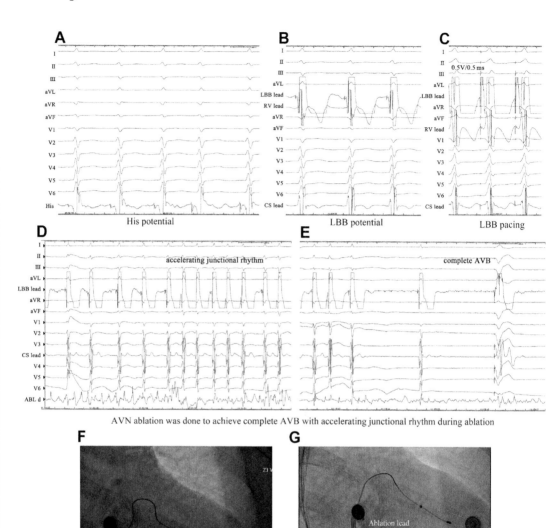

Fig. 9. Native ECG showed (*A*) His potential and (*B*) LBB potential; (*C*) LBB area pacing with LBBB correction; (*D*) accelerating junctional rhythm during ablation; (*E*) complete AV block occurred when AVN ablation achieved; (*F*) His lead; and (*G*) LBB area lead.

catheter (**Fig. 11**C). Then, a cryoablation catheter was used to achieve complete AV block (see **Fig. 11**B, D). After 2 years follow-up with HBP (**Fig. 11**E), cardiac function was improved from NYHA III to NYHA II.

Take-home messages:

1. Dilated cardiomyopathy with persistent AF case had an adequate rate-control by drug but severe HF symptoms persisted.

2. Cryoablation catheter was used to achieved AVN ablation while irrigated ablation catheter failed (see **Fig. 11**C, D).

Patient 8

A 56-year-old man with paroxysmal AF and congenital rupture of the inferior vena cava underwent surgical AF ablation in 2013. Afterward, he still presented with AF and repetitive acute HF

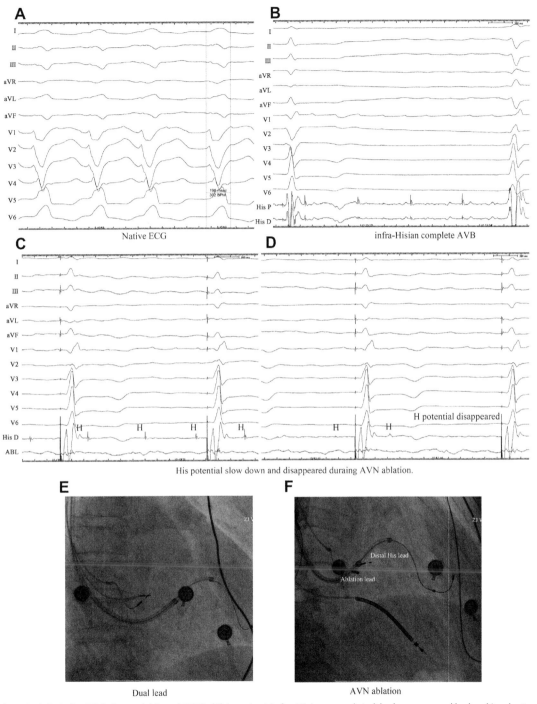

Fig. 10. (*A*) Native ECG showed AF and LBBB; (*B*) transient infra-Hisian complete block was caused by lead implantation; (*C, D*) reduction of rate and ultimate disappearance of His potential indicates successful AVN ablation; (*E*) fluoroscopic imaging of proximal and distal His lead; and (*F*) fluoroscopic imaging of ablation lead and his distal lead.

decompensation despite optimal drug therapy. The patient was referred for AVN ablation and pacemaker implantation in October 2017. At implantation, the lead was placed in the His region (**Fig. 12**D); His injury current was observed in His potential with H–V of 50 ms (**Fig. 12**A), His capture threshold of 0.9 V/0.5 ms (**Fig. 12**B), sensing amplitude of 9.5 mV, and impedance of 800 Ω. Additionally, another lead was placed in LBB region as a backup pacing (see **Fig. 12**E), with LBB potential to ventricular onset interval (LBBP-V) of 26 ms (**Fig. 12**A), LBB capture threshold of 0.4 V/

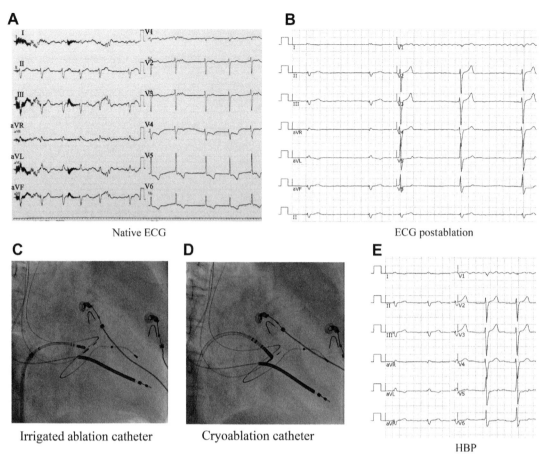

Fig. 11. (*A*) Native ECG showed AF; (*B*) ECG showed complete AV block postablation; fluoroscopic imaging showed the position of (*C*) cryoablation catheter and (*D*) irrigated ablation catheter; and (*E*) ECG showed narrow QRS with HBP.

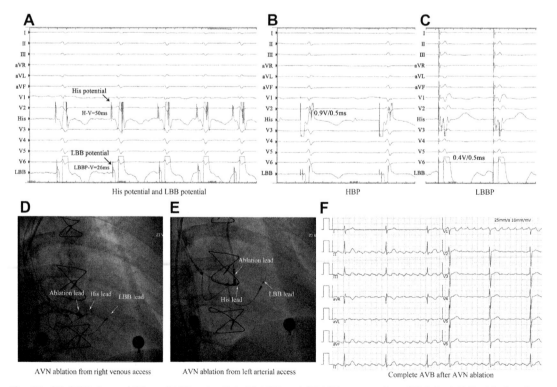

Fig. 12. (*A*) EGM showed His and LBB potential; (*B*) HBP and (*C*) LBB area pacing; (*D*) failed AVN ablation from venous access even close the His pacing site; (*E*) achieved AVN ablation through left arterial access; and (*F*) ECG showed complete AV block after AVN ablation.

0.5 ms (**Fig. 12**C), sensing amplitude of 9.4 mv, and impendence of 600 Ω. From right venous access, AVN ablation failed to achieve complete AV block at an ablating site close to the His pacing site (**Fig. 12**D). Finally, the authors obtained successful AVN ablation using left arterial access (**Fig. 12**E, F). Atrial lead was connected to A port, His lead was connected to RV port; LBB lead was connected to LV port (CRT-P, C2TR01, Medtronic).

Take-home messages:

1. Failed AVN ablation with venous access even close to the His pacing site was achieved through left arterial access (see **Fig. 12**D, E).
2. Dual leads: HBP and LBB area pacing (see **Fig. 12**D, E)

Summary of Take-Home Messages from These Cases

1. HBP combined with AVN ablation benefit AF patients with HF, especially for those with CRT nonresponse or suffer from ICD inappropriate shocks (case patients 2, 3, 4, and 8).
2. Pacing distal His bundle or bundle branch provides more operational space for AVN ablation (case patients 4, 5, and 6).
3. The dual lead method can be applied for alternately mapping and locating optimal pacing site (case patients 4, 6, and 8).
4. How to ablate the AVN when transient infra-Hisian complete block is caused by lead implantation (case patient 6).
5. How to rectify CLBBB without His potential recording (case patient 3)
6. AVN ablation through left arterial access and using cryoablation catheter (case patients 7 and 8)

SUMMARY AND PROSPECTS

Recently published literature shows that physiologic HBP coupled with AV node ablation could maintain the optimal ventricular synchrony. This therapeutic strategy is clinically safe and effective for HF patients with either permanent or paroxysmal AF, especially when the AF is the main cause of HF. AF ablation, however, should be considered as the first option for patients, especially younger patients, with paroxysmal AF, because these patients have the opportunity to maintain sinus rhythm after the procedure. Individual-based comprehensive and objective assessment is needed in the selection and recommendation of the treatment strategy. Because of the complexity of the procedure, it is recommended that the procedure should be conducted in centers with ample experience in electrophysiology and pacing therapy.

HBP is more physiologic compared with the RVP and BVP. By placing the lead to the distal of His bundle or even to the bundle branch, it is not only easier for ablating the AV node but also provides safer and stable pacing parameters. In the meantime, it may increase the probability of correcting typical CLBBB. At present, the clinical application of HBP is becoming more popular. The long-term safety issue has been addressed by pacing the distal area. Improvement of implant tools and more clinical research are warranted to confirm the great role of HBP combined with AVN ablation in AF patients with HF in the future.

ACKNOWLEDGEMENTS

This study was supported by Major Project of the Science and Technology of Wenzhou (ZS2017010).

REFERENCES

1. Chugh SS, Havmoeller R, Narayanan K, et al. Worldwide epidemiology of atrial fibrillation: a global burden of disease 2010 study. Circulation 2014; 129(8):837–47.
2. Heeringa J, van der Kuip DA, Hofman A, et al. Prevalence, incidence and lifetime risk of atrial fibrillation: the Rotterdam study. Eur Heart J 2006;27(8):949–53.
3. Lloyd-Jones DM, Wang TJ, Leip EP, et al. Lifetime risk for development of atrial fibrillation: the Framingham Heart Study. Circulation 2004;110(9):1042–6.
4. Benjamin EJ, Wolf PA, D'Agostino RB, et al. Impact of atrial fibrillation on the risk of death: the Framingham Heart Study. Circulation 1998;98(10):946–52.
5. Miyasaka Y, Barnes ME, Petersen RC, et al. Risk of dementia in stroke-free patients diagnosed with atrial fibrillation: data from a community-based cohort. Eur Heart J 2007;28(16):1962–7.
6. Anter E, Jessup M, Callans DJ. Atrial fibrillation and heart failure: treatment considerations for a dual epidemic. Circulation 2009;119(18):2516–25.
7. Hughes M, Lip GY, Guideline Development Group, National Clinical Guideline for Management of Atrial Fibrillation in Primary and Secondary Care, National Institute for Health and Clinical Excellence. Stroke and thromboembolism in atrial fibrillation: a systematic review of stroke risk factors, risk stratification schema and cost effectiveness data. Thromb Haemost 2008;99(2):295–304.
8. Abdul-Rahim AH, Perez AC, Fulton RL, et al. Risk of stroke in chronic heart failure patients without atrial fibrillation: analysis of the Controlled Rosuvastatin in Multinational Trial Heart Failure (CORONA) and the Gruppo Italiano per lo Studio della

Sopravvivenza nell'Insufficienza Cardiaca-Heart Failure (GISSI-HF) Trials. Circulation 2015;131(17): 1486–94 [discussion: 1494].

9. Savelieva I, Kakouros N, Kourliouros A, et al. Upstream therapies for management of atrial fibrillation: review of clinical evidence and implications for European Society of Cardiology guidelines. Part II: secondary prevention. Europace 2011;13(5):610–25.

10. Hagens VE, Van Veldhuisen DJ, Kamp O, et al. Effect of rate and rhythm control on left ventricular function and cardiac dimensions in patients with persistent atrial fibrillation: results from the RAte Control versus Electrical Cardioversion for Persistent Atrial Fibrillation (RACE) study. Heart Rhythm 2005;2(1):19–24.

11. Olshansky B, Heller EN, Mitchell LB, et al. Are transthoracic echocardiographic parameters associated with atrial fibrillation recurrence or stroke? Results from the Atrial Fibrillation Follow-Up Investigation of Rhythm Management (AFFIRM) study. J Am Coll Cardiol 2005;45(12):2026–33.

12. Bardy GH, Lee KL, Mark DB, et al. Amiodarone or an implantable cardioverter-defibrillator for congestive heart failure. N Engl J Med 2005; 352(3):225–37.

13. Kober L, Torp-Pedersen C, McMurray JJ, et al. Increased mortality after dronedarone therapy for severe heart failure. N Engl J Med 2008;358(25): 2678–87.

14. Chao TF, Liu CJ, Tuan TC, et al. Rate-control treatment and mortality in atrial fibrillation. Circulation 2015;132(17):1604–12.

15. Vamos M, Erath JW, Hohnloser SH. Digoxin-associated mortality: a systematic review and meta-analysis of the literature. Eur Heart J 2015;36(28):1831–8.

16. Mulder BA, Van Veldhuisen DJ, Crijns HJ, et al. Lenient vs. strict rate control in patients with atrial fibrillation and heart failure: a post-hoc analysis of the RACE II study. Eur J Heart Fail 2013;15(11):1311–8.

17. Khan MN, Jais P, Cummings J, et al. Pulmonary-vein isolation for atrial fibrillation in patients with heart failure. N Engl J Med 2008;359(17):1778–85.

18. MacDonald MR, Connelly DT, Hawkins NM, et al. Radiofrequency ablation for persistent atrial fibrillation in patients with advanced heart failure and severe left ventricular systolic dysfunction: a randomised controlled trial. Heart 2011;97(9):740–7.

19. Jones DG, Haldar SK, Hussain W, et al. A randomized trial to assess catheter ablation versus rate control in the management of persistent atrial fibrillation in heart failure. J Am Coll Cardiol 2013;61(18):1894–903.

20. Jons C, Hansen PS, Johannessen A, et al. The Medical ANtiarrhythmic Treatment or Radiofrequency Ablation in Paroxysmal Atrial Fibrillation (MANTRA-PAF) trial: clinical rationale, study design, and implementation. Europace 2009; 11(7):917–23.

21. Marrouche NF, Brachmann J, Andresen D, et al. Catheter ablation for atrial fibrillation with heart failure. N Engl J Med 2018;378(5):417–27.

22. Bhargava M, Di Biase L, Mohanty P, et al. Impact of type of atrial fibrillation and repeat catheter ablation on long-term freedom from atrial fibrillation: results from a multicenter study. Heart Rhythm 2009;6(10): 1403–12.

23. Marrouche NF, Wilber D, Hindricks G, et al. Association of atrial tissue fibrosis identified by delayed enhancement MRI and atrial fibrillation catheter ablation: the DECAAF study. JAMA 2014;311(5): 498–506.

24. Ganesan AN, Shipp NJ, Brooks AG, et al. Long-term outcomes of catheter ablation of atrial fibrillation: a systematic review and meta-analysis. J Am Heart Assoc 2013;2(2):e004549.

25. Wood MA, Brown-Mahoney C, Kay GN, et al. Clinical outcomes after ablation and pacing therapy for atrial fibrillation: a meta-analysis. Circulation 2000; 101(10):1138–44.

26. Tops LF, Schalij MJ, Holman ER, et al. Right ventricular pacing can induce ventricular dyssynchrony in patients with atrial fibrillation after atrioventricular node ablation. J Am Coll Cardiol 2006;48(8):1642–8.

27. Khurshid S, Epstein AE, Verdino RJ, et al. Incidence and predictors of right ventricular pacing-induced cardiomyopathy. Heart Rhythm 2014; 11(9):1619–25.

28. Doshi RN, Daoud EG, Fellows C, et al. Left ventricular-based cardiac stimulation post AV nodal ablation evaluation (the PAVE study). J Cardiovasc Electrophysiol 2005;16(11):1160–5.

29. Orlov MV, Gardin JM, Slawsky M, et al. Biventricular pacing improves cardiac function and prevents further left atrial remodeling in patients with symptomatic atrial fibrillation after atrioventricular node ablation. Am Heart J 2010;159(2):264–70.

30. Brignole M, Botto G, Mont L, et al. Cardiac resynchronization therapy in patients undergoing atrioventricular junction ablation for permanent atrial fibrillation: a randomized trial. Eur Heart J 2011; 32(19):2420–9.

31. Stavrakis S, Garabelli P, Reynolds DW. Cardiac resynchronization therapy after atrioventricular junction ablation for symptomatic atrial fibrillation: a meta-analysis. Europace 2012;14(10):1490–7.

32. Brignole M, Auricchio A, Baron-Esquivias G, et al. 2013 ESC guidelines on cardiac pacing and cardiac resynchronization therapy: the Task Force on cardiac pacing and resynchronization therapy of the European Society of Cardiology (ESC). Developed in collaboration with the European Heart Rhythm Association (EHRA). Eur Heart J 2013;34(29):2281–329.

33. January CT, Wann LS, Alpert JS, et al. 2014 AHA/ ACC/HRS guideline for the management of

patients with atrial fibrillation: a report of the American College of Cardiology/American Heart Association Task Force on Practice Guidelines and the Heart Rhythm Society. J Am Coll Cardiol 2014;64(21):e1–76.

34. Beshai JF, Grimm RA, Nagueh SF, et al. Cardiac-resynchronization therapy in heart failure with narrow QRS complexes. N Engl J Med 2007;357(24): 2461–71.

35. Ploux S, Eschalier R, Whinnett ZI, et al. Electrical dyssynchrony induced by biventricular pacing: implications for patient selection and therapy improvement. Heart Rhythm 2015;12(4):782–91.

36. Dandamudi G, Vijayaraman P. History of His bundle pacing. J Electrocardiol 2017;50(1):156–60.

37. Deshmukh P, Casavant DA, Romanyshyn M, et al. Permanent, direct His-bundle pacing: a novel approach to cardiac pacing in patients with normal His-Purkinje activation. Circulation 2000;101(8): 869–77.

38. Huang W, Su L, Wu S, et al. Benefits of permanent his bundle pacing combined with atrioventricular node ablation in atrial fibrillation patients with heart failure with both preserved and reduced left ventricular ejection fraction. J Am Heart Assoc 2017;6(4) [pii:e005309].

39. Vijayaraman P, Subzposh FA, Naperkowski A. Atrioventricular node ablation and His bundle pacing. Europace 2017;19(suppl_4):iv10–6.

40. Kirchhof P, Benussi S, Kotecha D, et al. 2016 ESC guidelines for the management of atrial fibrillation developed in collaboration with EACTS. Eur Heart J 2016;37(38):2893–962.

41. Vijayaraman P, Dandamudi G, Zanon F, et al. Permanent His bundle pacing: recommendations from a multicenter his bundle pacing collaborative working group for standardization of definitions, implant measurements, and follow-up. Heart Rhythm 2018; 15(3):460–8.

42. Teng AE, Lustgarten DL, Vijayaraman P, et al. Usefulness of his bundle pacing to achieve electrical resynchronization in patients with complete left bundle branch block and the relation between native QRS axis, duration, and normalization. Am J Cardiol 2016;118(4):527–34.

43. Lustgarten DL, Crespo EM, Arkhipova-Jenkins I, et al. His-bundle pacing versus biventricular pacing in cardiac resynchronization therapy patients: a crossover design comparison. Heart Rhythm 2015; 12(7):1548–57.

44. Shan P, Su L, Chen X, et al. Direct his-bundle pacing improved left ventricular function and remodelling in a biventricular pacing nonresponder. Can J Cardiol 2016;32(12):1577.e1–4.

45. Barba-Pichardo R, Morina-Vazquez P, Fernandez-Gomez JM, et al. Permanent His-bundle pacing: seeking physiological ventricular pacing. Europace 2010;12(4):527–33.

46. Wu G, Cai Y, Huang W, et al. Hisian pacing restores cardiac function. J Electrocardiol 2013;46(6):676–8.

47. Huang W, Su L, Wu S, et al. A novel pacing strategy with low and stable output: pacing the left bundle branch immediately beyond the conduction block. Can J Cardiol 2017;33(12):1736.e1–3.

48. Kulkarni N, Moore C, Pandey A, et al. His-bundle pacing for identifying optimal ablation sites in patients undergoing atrioventricular junction ablation. Pacing Clin Electrophysiol 2017;40(3):242–6.

49. Wang RX, Lee HC, Hodge DO, et al. Effect of pacing method on risk of sudden death after atrioventricular node ablation and pacemaker implantation in patients with atrial fibrillation. Heart Rhythm 2013; 10(5):696–701.

Long-Term Results of His Bundle Pacing

Faiz A. Subzposh, MD[a], Pugazhendhi Vijayaraman, MD, FHRS[a,b,c],*

KEYWORDS

- His bundle pacing • Right ventricular pacing • Heart failure hospitalization • Long-term outcomes

KEY POINTS

- His Bundle Pacing (HBP) is safe and feasible in the short-term.
- Long-term studies are few regarding HBP.
- Lead performance and clinical outcomes show promise in the long term.

INTRODUCTION

The number of patients requiring permanent pacemaker therapy has increased over the past several decades. The adverse effects of the early single-chamber pacemakers were quickly realized with regard to hemodynamics, and pacemakers that maintained atrioventricular (AV) synchrony were developed shortly afterward. Physiologic ventricular activation was then addressed with the advent of cardiac resynchronization therapy (CRT). His Bundle Pacing (HBP) is an alternative technique in pacing the ventricles "physiologically" that has shown promise in implant success and short-term follow-up,[1–3] especially with the advent of new lead technology and delivery mechanisms.

LONG-TERM OUTCOMES

The studies involving long-term outcomes of HBP are relatively few. A summary of the studies is published in **Table 1**. The first study that looked at HBP in humans involved patients with dilated cardiomyopathy and permanent atrial fibrillation (AF) by Deshmukh and colleagues.[4] HBP was performed in conjunction with AV node ablation.

Using a mapping catheter from the groin, His bundle pacing was performed to identify feasibility of selective capture. A fixed nonretractable screw-in lead was then advanced to that spot using "J"-shaped stylets and secured there. Eighty-six percent of these patients had successful HBP. Lead dislodgement was seen in 2 patients, one the day after and the other 2 months after implantation. Over a mean follow-up of 23 months, the investigators were able to show maintenance of HBP in 11 of 12 patients. Thresholds ranged from 2.4 ± 1.0 V at implant and increased to 3.9 ± 2.5 V at follow-up. Echocardiographic data also were measured in this study. Left ventricular ejection fraction (LV EF) and left ventricular end-diastolic diameter (LV EDD) improved in follow-up.

The same group of investigators published a study a few years later looking at a larger group of patients over a longer period of time.[5] Fifty-four patients who had permanent AF, dilated cardiomyopathy, and New York Heart Association (NYHA) Class III or IV were studied. Once again, a mapping catheter was used from the groin and a custom lead with a longer fixed helix was advanced using "J" stylets into the annulus area identified as the His region. Seventy-two percent

Disclosure: F.A. Subzposh - speaker (Medtronic); P. Vijayaraman – speaker, consultant, research (Medtronic), consultant (Abbott), advisory board (Boston Scientific).
[a] Cardiac Electrophysiology, Geisinger Heart Institute, MC 36-10, 1000 East Mountain Boulevard, Wilkes-Barre, PA 18711, USA; [b] Cardiac Electrophysiology, Geisinger Medical Center, Danville, PA, USA; [c] Geisinger Commonwealth School of Medicine, Scranton, PA, USA
* Corresponding author. Cardiac Electrophysiology, Geisinger Heart Institute, MC 36-10, 1000 East Mountain Boulevard, Wilkes-Barre, PA 18711.
E-mail addresses: pvijayaraman1@geisinger.edu; pvijayaraman@gmail.com

cardiacEP.theclinics.com

Table 1
Summary of His bundle pacing studies with medium to long-term follow-up

Author	No. of Patients	Success, %	Follow-up Duration, mo	Threshold, V	Sensing, mV	Impedance, ohms	Paced QRS, ms	LV EF, %
Deshmukh et al,[4] 2000	18	86	23	2.4 →3.9	1.7→2.2	488→723	92→104	18→28
Deshmukh et al,[5] 2004	54	72	42	—	—	—	—	23→33
Occhetta et al,[1] 2006	18	89	12	0.9 → 1	6.9 →	614 →	121 → similar	52→53
Kronburg et al,[6] 2014	34	84	24	1.0→1.5	—	—	—	—
Vijayaraman et al,[7] 2015	100	84	19	1.4→1.6	5.3→6.4	577→437	—	—
Huang et al,[8] 2017	52	80	21	1.1→1.2	3.5→3	—	—	44→64
Vijayaraman et al,[9] 2017	42	95	19	1→1.6	6→5.1	544→459	127→127	43→50
Vijayaraman et al,[10] 2017	20	—	70	1.9→2.5	5.9→6.1	516→484	117→118	50→55
Vijayaraman et al,[11] 2016	10	—	48	1.4→1.9	—	—	132→132	—
Zanon et al,[12] 2017	369	83	76	—	—	—	—	56→60
Vijayaraman et al,[13] 2018	94	80	60	1.4→1.6	6.8→7.2	639→463	122→126	55→57

Abbreviation: LV EF, left ventricular ejection fraction.

of patients were able to achieve selective HBP. Over a mean follow-up of 42 months, 10 patients died, and 2 generator replacement procedures were performed. Electrophysiological data were not reported. Patients showed improvement of their EF from 23% ± 11% to 33% ± 15%. Twelve of the patients had a His and right ventricular (RV) pacing lead placed and underwent cardiopulmonary testing that showed higher O_2 uptake with HBP compared with RV pacing from the apex. In 2006, Occhetta and colleagues[1] reported on the clinical advantage of para-Hisian pacing compared with RV pacing in 16 of 18 patients undergoing AV node ablation in a randomized, 6-month, crossover study. In this study, para-Hisian pacing resulted in improved interventricular mechanical delay, NYHA functional class, quality of life, 6-minute walk, and mitral and tricuspid regurgitation.

Kronburg and colleagues[6] randomized 34 patients to HBP or RV pacing for a period of 12 months each and followed them clinically in a double-blind, crossover study. All patients had AV block with approximately 99% ventricular pacing. The EF with RV pacing was significantly lower than with HBP. Thresholds rose significantly from 1.0 V to 1.5 V and 1 patient developed exit block after 15 months.

In 2015, Vijayaraman and colleagues[7] published a study involving 100 patients with advanced AV block followed over a mean of 19 months. Success rate of HBP was 84% using the Select Secure (Model 3830, Medtronic Inc, Minneapolis, MN) lead delivered through a fixed curve sheath (C315 His, Medtronic Inc). Pacing thresholds at implant were reported as 1.4 ± 1.0 V and increased to 1.6 ± 1.0 V at follow-up. Impedance values and sensed R waves remained stable in the follow-up period. Five percent of patients had a significant increase in their pacing threshold requiring revision or replacement. This occurred in 2 weeks in 2 patients and between 2 months and 6 months in the remaining 3 patients. Patients were further divided into those with AV nodal block (normal QRS) and those with infranodal block (wide QRS). The 2 groups had similar outcomes in follow-up.

In 2017, Huang and colleagues[8] published a study looking at HBP in patients with symptomatic AF requiring AV nodal ablation. Fifty-two patients were attempted with 81% implant success. These patients were followed for a mean of 21 months looking at echocardiographic changes as well as clinical outcomes. One patient required a generator change during the follow-up period. Despite all patients having had hospitalizations for heart failure within 1 year of the procedure, only 2 patients (4.8%) had heart failure–related admissions after HBP. There were 5 patients who had a significant change in their pacing threshold (>1 V). In the remaining patients, thresholds as well as sensing and impedances remained stable. Echocardiographic data also showed improvement in their LV EF as well as LV EDD. The magnitude of improvement significantly correlated to the baseline severity of ventricular dysfunction.

Another study looking at a similar patient population was published by Vijayaraman and colleagues.[9] The study involved 42 patients undergoing AV node ablation and HBP, followed over a mean of 19 months with a 95% success rate of HBP. One patient needed lead revision due to acute threshold rise. Five patients died in follow-up (non–lead-related deaths) as well as 3 patients (7%) had heart failure hospitalizations. Lead parameters remained relatively stable in follow-up. Thresholds were 1.0 ± 0.8 V at implant and rose to 1.6 ± 1.2 V at follow-up. Echocardiographic data showed improvement of EF from a mean of 43% to 50%. Most of the improvement was seen in patients with an EF less than 40% similar to findings reported by Huang and colleagues.[8]

In assessing whether HBP caused or worsened existing His-Purkinje conduction disease in long-term follow-up, Vijayaraman and his colleagues[10] published a study looking at 20 patients who presented for generator change with HBP. At the time of generator change, His capture threshold and HV intervals were measured as well as incremental pacing from the lead at 700, 600, and 500 ms was done to assess for 1:1 capture of the conduction system. Mean duration of HBP at generator change was 70 months. Two patients had admissions for heart failure hospitalizations in that time period. Paced QRS, sensed R waves, and pacing impedances were similar to implant values (Fig. 1). His capture thresholds were 1.9 ± 1.1 V at implant and rose significantly to 2.5 ± 1.2 V at the time of generator change. HV intervals did not change significantly and all patients tested showed a 1:1 capture pacing at 500 ms through the pacing lead, allowing the investigators to conclude that no significant progression of His-Purkinje conduction disease had occurred in these patients. Echocardiographic data showed improvement from a mean of 50% at implant to

55% at the time of generator change as well as a decrease in LV EDD.

Another study supporting this idea of HBP not accelerating His-Purkinje conduction disease was done by Vijayaraman and colleagues[11] looking at patients with intra-Hisian block. Patients with intra-Hisian conduction block whose QRS morphologies were abnormal at baseline but could be normalized with HBP were included in the study. Ten patients were followed for 4 years, with 1 patient needing a lead revision at 2 weeks due to high threshold. Pacing thresholds were 1.4 ± 1.2 V at implant and increased to 1.9 ± 1.0 V at follow-up. All patients had persistently narrow QRS during follow-up. The investigators of the abstract were able to conclude from the stable HBP thresholds and QRS morphologies that in 4 years' time, intra-Hisian block had not progressed.

Zanon and colleagues[12] retrospectively analyzed 344 patients over a mean of 76 months. Eighty-three percent of patients showed successful HBP at end of follow-up with similar QRS morphologies compared with implantation. Mean thresholds at follow-up were 2.6 ± 1.6 V, although implant values were not reported. Five patients required upgrade to biventricular pacing and 188 patients required generator change due to battery depletion. Heart failure episodes were reported in only 8% of these patients.

The most recent study looking at 5-year follow-up was published by Vijayaraman and colleagues.[13] HBP was attempted in 94 consecutive patients requiring permanent pacemakers and was successful in 80% of patients. Five patients required lead revisions: 2 patients at 2 weeks due to high threshold; 1 patient required revision at 2 years due to increased threshold >5 V; 2 patients had lead revision at time of generator change due to high thresholds. Over 5 years, pacing thresholds significantly increased from 1.35 ± 0.9 V to 1.62 ± 1.0 V. Sensing R waves remained stable and pacing impedances significantly dropped from 639 ± 159 Ω to 463 ± 78 Ω. Seven patients required generator change due to battery depletion. Pacing-induced cardiomyopathy was noted in 22% of RV-paced patients compared with 2% in the HBP group (P<.01). Paced QRS morphologies and durations remained stable, with HBP suggesting no evidence of progression to distal His-Purkinje conduction disease.

This study compared outcomes of HBP with a similar cohort of patients receiving RV pacing. When on-treatment analysis was performed (n = 75), there was a significantly increased risk of combined endpoint of death or Heart failure hospitalization in the RV pacing (41% vs 27%;

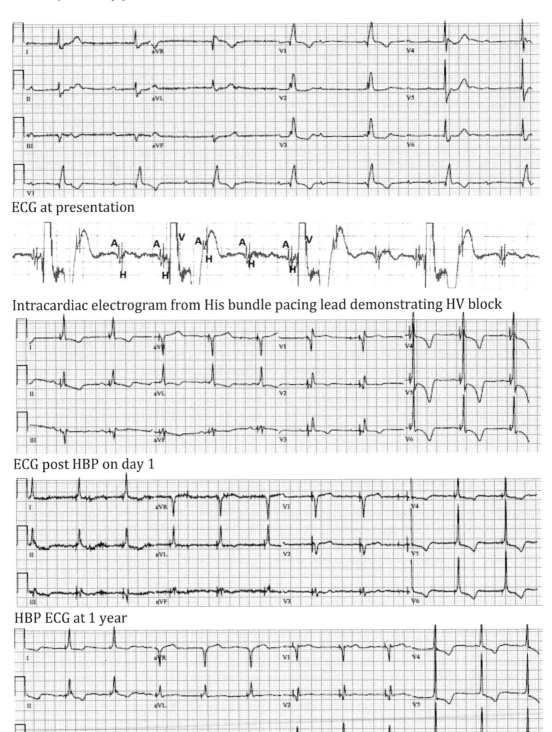

ECG at presentation

Intracardiac electrogram from His bundle pacing lead demonstrating HV block

ECG post HBP on day 1

HBP ECG at 1 year

ECG at the time of pacemaker generator change at 6 years

Fig. 1. Electrocardiograms (ECGs) of HBP. Twelve-lead ECG during presentation with complete heart block along with intracardiac electrograms recorded from the HBP lead (showing HV block) are shown along with ECGs during HBP at 1 day, 1 year, and 6 years after implant. The paced QRS morphology and duration remained similar during follow-up. T-wave memory changes noted immediately after HBP resolved during follow-up. His capture threshold was 2 V at 1 ms at implant and increased to 2.5 V at 1 ms during follow-up and remained stable thereafter up to 6 years.

hazard ratio [HR] 1.7; $P = .04$) group compared with the HBP group during the 5-year follow-up (**Fig. 2**). When further looking at patients with greater than 40% ventricular pacing, this disparity between groups was even greater. When looking at intention-to-treat analysis in the 2 groups with greater than 40% ventricular pacing, including the patients with failed HBP, there was significant difference in the combined outcomes in the 5-year follow-up.

DISCUSSION

There are few studies looking at long-term outcomes related to HBP. In those described previously, the Medtronic 3830 lead was used in most. This lead, released in 2005, shortened procedure time, as well as allowed operators to easily find the His bundle region and often without the need for a mapping catheter. This overall led to adaption of HBP in more centers. Most of the studies quote both acute and chronic increase in His capture thresholds. It is unclear at this time whether it is related to lead design (fixed screw with steroid coating) or related to the anatomy of the His bundle and its proximity to the tricuspid annulus, which will cause the lead tip to experience stress due to valve motion. Additionally, a higher incidence of lead revisions (~5%) is required in patients undergoing permanent HBP. It is necessary to understand the mechanisms involved in threshold increases and need for lead revision and consider changes in lead design and delivery systems.

Using HBP to correct bundle branch delay or block is feasible but not perfect. In the study by Vijayaraman and colleagues,[7] HBP was successful in 76% of patients with infranodal block compared with 93% success rate in patients with AV nodal block. This difference may be related to underlying pathology and difficulty in accessing the distal His bundle. In the medium-term follow-up of 4 to 6 years, the paced QRS morphology and His-Purkinje conduction remained relatively stable without progression[10,11]; however, much needs to be learned regarding the safety and stability of HBP during longer term.

Although there are no long-term randomized studies assessing clinical outcomes of HBP compared with RV pacing, one observational study has shown promise for reduction in combined endpoint of heart failure hospitalization and mortality.[13] In comparing HBP with RV pacing, most of the benefit was seen in patients with higher ventricular pacing burden. This endorses the theory of HBP as the best option for electrical and hemodynamic benefit in those needing ventricular pacing. Most of the studies reporting on LV EF showed no significant decrease and an improvement when HBP was used in patients with cardiomyopathy. Currently there are very few ongoing randomized clinical trials assessing the use of HBP when compared with CRT in patients with cardiomyopathy. Long-term randomized clinical studies are essential to fully evaluate the safety and durability of HBP and to prove the observed and perceived improved clinical outcomes in patients requiring permanent HBP. If

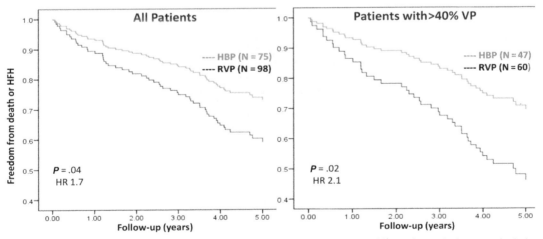

Fig. 2. Clinical outcomes of HBP compared with RV pacing. Cox proportional hazards survival curves depicting combined endpoint of death or heart failure hospitalization comparing HBP with RV pacing in all patients and those with greater than 40% ventricular pacing. RVP, right ventricular pacing; VP, ventricular pacing burden. (*Data from* Vijayaraman P, Naperkowski A, Subzposh FA, et al. Permanent His bundle pacing: long-term lead performance and clinical outcomes. Heart Rhythm 2018;15(5):696–702.)

clinical trials confirm these benefits, and improvements in lead and delivery tools are achieved, it is likely that HBP will become the physiologic pacing site of choice.

REFERENCES

1. Occhetta E, Bortnik M, Magnani A, et al. Prevention of ventricular desynchronization by permanent para-hisian pacing after atrioventricular node ablation in chronic atrial fibrillation: a crossover, blinded randomized study versus right ventricular pacing. J Am Coll Cardiol 2006;47:1938–45.

2. Zanon F, Baracca E, Aggio S, et al. A feasible approach for direct His bundle pacing using a new steerable catheter to facilitate precise lead placement. J Cardiovasc Electrophysiol 2006;17:29–33.

3. Zanon F, Svetlich C, Occhetta E, et al. Safety and performance of a system specifically designed for selective site pacing. Pacing Clin Electrophysiol 2011;34:339–47.

4. Deshmukh P, Casavant D, Romanyshyn M, et al. Permanent, direct His-bundle pacing: a novel approach to cardiac pacing in patients with normal His-Purkinje activation. Circulation 2000;101:869–77.

5. Deshmukh P, Romanyshyn M. Direct His-bundle pacing. Pacing Clin Electrophysiol 2004;27:862–70.

6. Kronburg M, Mortensen PT, Poulsen SH, et al. His or para-His pacing preserves left ventricular function in atrioventricular block: a double-blind, randomized, crossover study. Europace 2014;16:1189–96.

7. Vijayaraman P, Naperkowski A, Ellenbogen KA, et al. Electrophysiologic insights into site of atrioventricular block: lessons from permanent His bundle pacing. JACC Clin Electrophysiol 2015;1:571–81.

8. Huang W, Su L, Wu S, et al. Benefits of permanent His bundle pacing combined with atrioventricular node ablation in atrial fibrillation patients with heart failure with both preserved and reduced left ventricular ejection fraction. J Am Heart Assoc 2017;6: e005309.

9. Vijayaraman P, Subzposh F, Naperkowski A. Atrioventricular node ablation and His bundle pacing. Europace 2017;19:iv10–6.

10. Vijayaraman P, Dandamudi G, Lustgarten D, et al. Permanent His bundle pacing: electrophysiological and echocardiographic observations from long-term follow-up. Pacing Clin Electrophysiol 2017;7: 883–91.

11. Vijayaraman P, Dandamudi G. Intra-Hisian block: stable distal His-Purkinje conduction at 4 years during permanent His bundle pacing [abstract]. Heart Rhythm 2016;13:S147.

12. Zanon F, Marcantoni L, Pastore G, et al. P1351Long-term follow-up of His pacing in a single center experience [abstract]. Eur Heart J 2017;38:ehx502. P1351.

13. Vijayaraman P, Naperkowski A, Subzposh FA, et al. Permanent His bundle pacing: long-term lead performance and clinical outcomes. Heart Rhythm 2018;15(5):696–702.

Future Developments in His Bundle Pacing

Harsimran Saini, MD, PhD, Kenneth A. Ellenbogen, MD*, Jayanthi N. Koneru, MBBS

KEYWORDS

• His bundle pacing • Clinical trials • Future developments

KEY POINTS

• Because there has been a significant push toward His bundle pacing (HBP), multiple studies and advancements are underway to provide new and improved delivery tools and lead designs, allowing one to apply this technology in daily practice.
• A better understanding of the pacing configurations and ultimately development of dedicated algorithms will alleviate some of these aforementioned challenges.
• Ultimately, with such technological advances and mounting clinical evidence, one can surely anticipate HBP to revolutionize the field of cardiac pacing.

INTRODUCTION

The past few decades have seen significant advances in cardiac implantable electronic device therapies. A continually increasing emphasis on the study of electrophysiological mechanisms has driven the field of cardiac electrophysiology. Recently, there has been resurgence in the concept of physiologic pacing using the His Purkinje system, which has emerged as an alternative solution to traditional right ventricular (RV) pacing as well as resynchronization therapy.

The observations by Purkinje and His and the seminal work of Sunao Tawara established the framework and paved the way for the future investigations into the cardiac conduction system. In 1919, Kaufman and Rothberger first conceptualized the functional longitudinal dissociation of His bundle. They were the first to propose that normal conduction in the His Purkinje system was mediated by pathways originating in the atrioventricular (AV) junction that connected to predesignated right or left ventricular Purkinje fibers. In 1977, Narula[1] demonstrated in a series on 27 patients with left bundle branch block (LBBB) and prolonged His-ventricular (HV) intervals, the ability to normalize the QRS complex with His-bundle pacing (HBP). Then, in 1978, El-Sherif and colleagues[2] showed that in patients with acute right bundle branch block (RBBB) after a myocardial infarction and those with chronic LBBB, His bundle-pacing resulted in normalization of the QRS complex with a shorter stimulus to ventricular interval compared with the intrinsic HV interval, likely because of the site of pacing being distal to the location of block.[3] Deshmukh and colleagues[4] were the first to study the immediate and long-term effects of HBP in patients who had heart failure, atrial fibrillation (AF), and AV nodal ablation; they showed an improvement in the left ventricular ejection fraction (LVEF), decreased left ventricular (LV) dimensions, and improved clinical outcomes.

This article provides a summary of the recent studies in the field of HBP as well as ongoing clinical trials and future developments.

HIS BUNDLE PACING: A PHYSIOLOGIC WAY OF PACING THE HEART

HBP can be advantageous in patients with conduction disease without heart failure. As demonstrated by DAVID I and DAVID II trials, a high

VCU School of Medicine, Medical College of Virginia Hospitals, Richmond, VA, USA
* Corresponding author. Division of Cardiovascular Diseases, Virginia Commonwealth University Health Science Center, 1200 East Marshall Street, Gateway Building, 3rd Floor, 3-216, Richmond, VA 232980053.
E-mail address: Kenneth.Ellenbogen@vcuhealth.org

Card Electrophysiol Clin 10 (2018) 543–548
https://doi.org/10.1016/j.ccep.2018.05.013
1877-9182/18/© 2018 Elsevier Inc. All rights reserved.

percentage of RV pacing induces a similar level of dyssynchrony and shares similar outcomes to patients with heart failure and LBBB, including an increased risk of AF and death.[5,6] Biventricular (Biv) pacing mitigates such detrimental effects of RV-only pacing. The BLOCK-HF study demonstrated superiority of Biv to RV-only pacing and showed a significant mortality benefit and improved clinical outcomes with improved New York Heart Association (NYHA) class as well as quality of life. Furthermore, Biv pacing resulted in reverse remodeling as demonstrated by improved echocardiographic indices.[7]

HBP similarly mitigates the adverse effects of RV-only pacing and was shown to be associated with significantly lower heart failure hospitalizations.[8] In a long-term follow-up study, despite high pacing burden, patients with a His bundle pacemaker had a stable LVEF, suggesting long-lasting benefits of HBP.[9] A recent study by Huang and colleagues[10] studied 52 patients with heart failure and narrow QRS, who underwent AV node ablation for AF and received His bundle pacemakers. In the postablation period, patients with HBP had significantly improved LVEF, LV end diastolic pressure, and NYHA functional status as well as decreased diuretic use. These clinical benefits were of greater magnitude in patients with reduced LVEF.

Heart failure with impaired left ventricular function with conduction abnormalities is an ominous combination that results in ventricular dyssynchrony, further decline of heart function, and an increased risk of death.[11] Cardiac resynchronization therapy (CRT) is established as a treatment of systolic HF with ventricular dyssynchrony as described by the presence of an LBBB with QRS greater than 140 milliseconds.[12–15] To date, multiple studies have demonstrated improved mortality, left ventricular function, and quality of life in patients with reduced LVEF and LBBB who undergo CRT.[15,16] As such, CRT has become a guideline-recommended therapy. However, CRT achieved with Biv pacing can be mired with multiple challenges. Occasionally, natural anatomic vein variations preclude feasibility of delivering the CS lead successfully, and even when the lead is delivered successfully, the nonresponse rate for CRT can be as high as 30%.[17,18] In addition, the site of latest activation in the left ventricle might not be accessible for lead delivery. Moreover, functional lines of block occur in patients with underlying heart block and RV pacing. Currently, the only way to identify the latest site of activation in this situation is via activation mapping and 3-dimensional electroanatomical mapping. Furthermore, the added risks of CS

dissection/perforation during implantation and reversed depolarization and repolarization sequence due to epicardial pacing pose additional risks to patients. Although challenges exist with HBP also, even in its early stages, it appears to be an attractive and safe alternative. Since the early works by Deshmukh and colleagues,[4] several studies have provided sufficient evidence in support of using HBP in the treatment of conduction abnormalities as well as in patients with heart failure.

HIS BUNDLE PACING AS AN ALTERNATIVE TO BIVENTRICULAR CARDIAC RESYNCHRONIZATION THERAPY

Sharma and colleagues[19] recently reported that the HBP in 2 CRT nonresponders significantly narrowed the QRS interval (165 ± 31 to 115 ± 13 milliseconds) and improved the LVEF (30 ± 10 to 47 ± 11%) and NYHA functional class. A study by Shan and colleagues[20] demonstrated similar results in a CRT nonresponder patient. Several studies have reported the use of HBP for CRT with success rates ranging from 56% to 92%. Barba-Pichardo and colleagues[21] reported a 56% success rate in HBP among cardiomyopathy patients with failed CRT with improvements in NYHA class and LVEF. Lustgarten and colleagues[22] performed a randomized crossover patient-blinded study comparing CRT and HBP in patients meeting CRT indications. After an initial assignment to either group, patients were crossed over to the other group after 6 months and followed for another 6 months. The study reported a 72% success rate with HBP for CRT, with clinical improvements in 6-minute walk, NYHA functional class, quality of life, and LVEF in both CRT and HBP arms. HBP in lieu of an LV lead is also feasible. Ajijola and colleagues[23] recently reported significant QRS narrowing, improved NYHA functional class, and LV dimensions in 21 patients with an indication for CRT. HBP is a possible alternative to CRT for systolic HF and conduction delay. A recent study published by Sharma and colleagues[19] assessing HBP for CRT in CRT-eligible patients and CRT nonresponders further showed the feasibility of HBP for CRT. The study reported a 90% success rate with significant QRS narrowing (157 ± 33 to 117 ± 18 milliseconds), increase in LVEF, and improvement in NYHA class after 14-month follow-up. Furthermore, HBP may also provide an opportunity for patients with RBBB or nonspecific interventricular conduction delay.[19] Vijayaraman and colleagues[8] demonstrated QRS narrowing in 94% of patients (29 of 31) with

RBBB and 20% of patients (1 of 5) in with ICVD. Sharma and colleagues[24] included 12/106 (11%) patients with non-LBBB with overall successful narrowing of QRS in 90% of cases attempted.

The studies listed above only underscore the importance of HBP as the next frontier in pacing and cardiac resynchronization therapies. Several clinical trials and studies are underway to further optimize the ways in which one approaches and performs HBP.

Although there are no data on patients who have complete heart block and *no underlying rhythm* after cardiac surgery, HBP has been safely accomplished using *pace mapping* at the putative site of interest (**Fig. 1**). There is a need for these patients to be included in future studies, given the increasing number of percutaneous as well as open chest valve surgeries.

ONGOING CLINICAL TRIALS

The results from 3 ongoing randomized clinical trials comparing HBP and Biv-CRT (His-SYNC NCT02700425, HOPE-HF, and NCT02805465) will likely add to what is known about HBP and CRT. His-SYNC is a randomized clinical trial and is currently enrolling heart failure patients eligible for CRT and evaluating the efficacy of HBP versus conventional BiV-CRT. HOPE-HF is also currently enrolling with randomized crossover arms of no pacing versus HBP in HF patients. A comparison was made between HBP and BiV pacing in HF patients with AF who need an AVN ablation (NCT02805465) in a randomized, crossover, double-blinded study comparing HBP and BiV pacing currently recruiting participants in HF patients with AF. **Table 1** summarizes the ongoing clinical trials as listed on clinicaltrials.gov that are underway to further investigate the mechanisms and clinical efficacy of HBP.

Image-HBP is a multicenter prospective trial, with a proposed sample size of approximately 60 patients, that will focus on assessing the lead electrical measurements on implantation, determine changes over time, and estimate the correlation between lead location and selective versus nonselective HBP. The purpose of this study is to estimate the correlation between long-term lead performance and implant characteristics (NCT03294317). Perioperative chest computed tomography will be performed and is expected to provide information to characterize the precise location and relationship of the lead to the tricuspid annulus, right atrium, right ventricle, and interventricular and AV septum.

The role of HBP in bradycardia and heart failure is being evaluated in an observational study. The investigators intend to test the effects of selective versus nonselective HBP in patients with heart failure with regard to narrowing of the QRS complex and improvement of AV conduction in functional bundle branch block or conduction delay (NCT03008291). Another ongoing randomized control study aims to compare direct HBP with

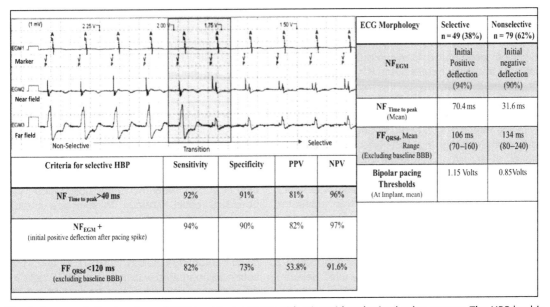

ECG Morphology	Selective n = 49 (38%)	Nonselective n = 79 (62%)
NF$_{EGM}$	Initial Positive deflection (94%)	Initial negative deflection (90%)
NF $_{Time\ to\ peak}$ (Mean)	70.4 ms	31.6 ms
FF$_{QRSd}$ Mean Range (Excluding baseline BBB)	106 ms (70–160)	134 ms (80–240)
Bipolar pacing Thresholds (At Implant, mean)	1.15 Volts	0.85 Volts

Criteria for selective HBP	Sensitivity	Specificity	PPV	NPV
NF $_{Time\ to\ peak}$ >40 ms	92%	91%	81%	96%
NF$_{EGM}$ + (initial positive deflection after pacing spike)	94%	90%	82%	97%
FF $_{QRSd}$ <120 ms (excluding baseline BBB)	82%	73%	53.8%	91.6%

Fig. 1. Representative location of HBP lead in a patient with tricuspid and mitral valve surgery. The HBP lead is distal and septal to the tricuspid valve ring. Also shown in the figure is the 12-lead electrocardiogram (ECG), which demonstrates HBP achieved purely by pace mapping because this patient had AF and no ventricular escape. NPV, negative predictive value; PPV, positive predictive value.

Table 1
Summary of the ongoing clinical trials as listed on clinicaltrials.gov that are underway to further investigate the mechanisms and clinical efficacy of His bundle pacing

Clinical Trial Designation	Study Title	Study Design
NCT02671903	The His Optimized Pacing Evaluated for Heart Failure Trial (HOPE-HF)	Multicenter double-blinded randomized control trial with 160 patients
NCT03452462	Electrical Resynchronization and Acute Hemodynamic Effects of Direct His Bundle Pacing Compared to Biventricular Pacing	Single-center, randomized clinical trial involving approximately 20 patients
NCT03294317	Imaging Study of Lead Implant for His Bundle Pacing (IMAGE-HBP)	Multicenter, observation study of 55 patients
NCT02805465	Comparison of His Bundle Pacing and Bi-Ventricular Pacing in Heart Failure with Atrial Fibrillation	Multicenter, prospective, randomized crossover study of 50 patients
NCT02700425	His Bundle Pacing vs Coronary Sinus Pacing for Cardiac Resynchronization Therapy	Multicenter randomized, single-blinded study of 40 patients
NCT03008291	His Bundle Pacing in Bradycardia and Heart Failure	Single-center observational study of 40 patients

Biv pacing in terms of electrical resynchronization using electrocardiographic imaging. The study will weigh the effects on acute hemodynamic changes using finger plethysmography and conduction velocimetry.

FUTURE DEVELOPMENTS

Significant advances have been made with regards to implanting His bundle pacemakers with advent of selective lead delivery systems that are routinely used in daily practice. From the technical perspective, one must understand the intricate anatomic details of the His bundle region. The complex anatomy of this region can pose technical challenges of lead stability and design. First, the His bundle shares a close relationship with the membranous septum, and thus unlike a diagnostic catheter, the HBP lead must be positioned at an orthogonal angle into a region with minimal trabeculations. For clinicians, these factors often lead to prolonged procedural as well as fluoroscopy times. However, this presents unique opportunities for catheter and sheath designs. Currently, there are preformed (C315; Medtronic Inc, Minneapolis, MN, USA) as well as a deflectable sheath (C304; Medtronic Inc) that allows delivery of the most commonly used Select-Secure 3830 lead (Medtronic Inc).[25] Despite novel sheath delivery systems, there continues to be a need for sheaths that will tackle the issues of right-sided device implantations and are currently in the works.

Clinicians often use anatomic structures as markers under fluoroscopy to aid in optimal localization of the His bundle. In certain cases, a standard diagnostic electrophysiology catheter can be used as a fluoroscopic marker while placing the HBP lead.[26] Preexisting prosthetic valves can also serve as fluoroscopic aids. Sharma and colleagues[27] showed that successful HBP sites were posterior and inferior to aortic valve prosthetic rings/stents and distal and septal to the tricuspid valve ring, with overall success rate of 93%. With regards to procedural fluoroscopy times, Narula[1] initially reported mean procedural time of 3.7 ± 1.6 hours, which in subsequent studies from 2015 had improved to 64 ± 10 minutes with total fluoroscopy time of 8.9 ± 4 minutes.[28,29]

High capture thresholds can be encountered with HBP, considering that the His bundle region is surrounded by fibrous tissue. Despite that, multiple studies have suggested that capture thresholds are comparable to LV pacing and remain stable over time.[30,31] Recently, Su and colleagues[32] proposed a novel strategy to minimize capture threshold in His bundle pacemakers by using integrated bipolar configuration (His tip-RV coil). They showed that integrated bipolar pacing resulted in lower capture thresholds (1.13 ± 0.51 V at 0.5 milliseconds) compared with unipolar (1.75 ± 0.83 V at 0.5 milliseconds) and bipolar tip-ring (1.59 ± 0.71 V at 0.5 milliseconds).

In order to enhance battery longevity, as well as to identify the effective delivery of HBP, electrophysiologic principles that compare near-field

POST TRICUSPID AND MITRAL VALVE SURGERY WITH NO UNDERLYING RHYTHM

LAO   RAO   12 lead Electrocardiogram

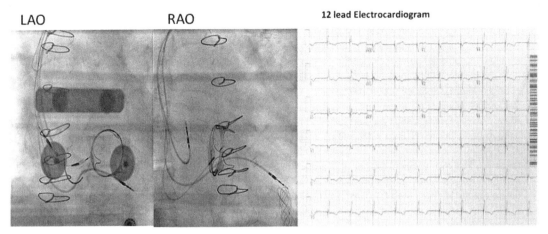

Fig. 2. An initial positive NF_{EGM} was frequently seen with S-HBP as opposed to negative in NS-HBP cases. A positive NF_{EGM} and $NF_{Time\ to\ peak}$ greater than 40 milliseconds were highly sensitive and specific for S-HBP irrespective of baseline QRSd or BBB patterns. Although FF_{QRSd} <120 milliseconds (patients with narrow QRS) was not as sensitive or specific, all 3 parameters had excellent negative predictive value. Morphologic transitions were correlated prospectively in 12 patients. As depicted in the figure, a clear transition in NF_{EGM} is noted correlating with a change from NS-HBP to S-HBP on simultaneous ECG. FF, far field; LAO, left anterior oblique; NF, Near Field; NS-HBP, non-selective HBP; RAO, right anterior oblique; S-HBP, selective-HBP.

and far-field electrograms can be used to develop automatic capture algorithms for HBP and to detect percent pacing-analogous to effective Biv pacing (**Fig. 2**).[33]

Because there has been a significant push toward HBP, multiple studies and advancements are underway to provide new and improved delivery tools and lead designs allowing one to apply this technology in daily practice. A better understanding of the pacing configurations and ultimately development of dedicated algorithms will alleviate some of these aforementioned challenges. Ultimately, with such technological advances and mounting clinical evidence, one can surely anticipate HBP to revolutionize the field of cardiac pacing.

REFERENCES

1. Narula OS. Longitudinal dissociation in the His bundle. Bundle branch block due to asynchronous conduction within the His bundle in man. Circulation 1977;56(6):996–1006.
2. El-Sherif N, Amay YLF, Schonfield C, et al. Normalization of bundle branch block patterns by distal His bundle pacing. Clinical and experimental evidence of longitudinal dissociation in the pathologic his bundle. Circulation 1978;57(3):473–83.
3. Scherlag BJ, El-Sherif N, Hope RR, et al. The significance of dissociation of conduction in the canine His bundle. Electrophysiological studies in vivo and in vitro. J Electrocardiol 1978;11(4):343–54.
4. Deshmukh P, Casavant DA, Romanyshyn M, et al. Permanent, direct His-bundle pacing: a novel approach to cardiac pacing in patients with normal His-Purkinje activation. Circulation 2000;101(8): 869–77.
5. Wilkoff BL, Cook JR, Epstein AE, et al. Dual-chamber pacing or ventricular backup pacing in patients with an implantable defibrillator: the Dual Chamber and VVI Implantable Defibrillator (DAVID) Trial. JAMA 2002;288(24):3115–23.
6. Wilkoff BL, Kudenchuk PJ, Buxton AE, et al. The DAVID (Dual Chamber and VVI Implantable Defibrillator) II trial. J Am Coll Cardiol 2009;53(10):872–80.
7. Curtis AB, Worley SJ, Chung ES, et al. Improvement in clinical outcomes with biventricular versus right ventricular pacing: the BLOCK HF study. J Am Coll Cardiol 2016;67(18):2148–57.
8. Sharma PS, Dandamudi G, Naperkowski A, et al. Permanent His-bundle pacing is feasible, safe, and superior to right ventricular pacing in routine clinical practice. Heart Rhythm 2015;12(2):305–12.
9. Vijayaraman P, Dandamudi G, Lustgarten D, et al. Permanent his bundle pacing: electrophysiological and echocardiographic observations from long-term follow-up. Pacing Clin Electrophysiol 2017; 40(7):883–91.
10. Huang W, Su L, Wu S, et al. Benefits of permanent his bundle pacing combined with atrioventricular node ablation in atrial fibrillation patients with heart failure with both preserved and reduced left ventricular ejection fraction. J Am Heart Assoc 2017;6(4) [pii:e005309].

11. Bleeker GB, Schalij MJ, Molhoek SG, et al. Relationship between QRS duration and left ventricular dyssynchrony in patients with end-stage heart failure. J Cardiovasc Electrophysiol 2004;15(5):544–9.

12. Bristow MR, Saxon LA, Boehmer J, et al. Cardiac-resynchronization therapy with or without an implantable defibrillator in advanced chronic heart failure. N Engl J Med 2004;350(21):2140–50.

13. Cleland JG, Daubert JC, Erdmann E, et al. The effect of cardiac resynchronization on morbidity and mortality in heart failure. N Engl J Med 2005;352(15):1539–49.

14. Moss AJ, Hall WJ, Cannom DS, et al. Cardiac-resynchronization therapy for the prevention of heart-failure events. N Engl J Med 2009;361(14):1329–38.

15. Epstein AE, DiMarco JP, Ellenbogen KA, et al. 2012 ACCF/AHA/HRS focused update incorporated into the ACCF/AHA/HRS 2008 guidelines for device-based therapy of cardiac rhythm abnormalities: a report of the American College of Cardiology Foundation/American Heart Association Task Force on Practice Guidelines and the Heart Rhythm Society. Circulation 2013;127(3):e283–352.

16. Gasparini M, Leclercq C, Yu CM, et al. Absolute survival after cardiac resynchronization therapy according to baseline QRS duration: a multinational 10-year experience: data from the Multicenter International CRT Study. Am Heart J 2014;167(2):203–9.e1.

17. Yu CM, Hayes DL. Cardiac resynchronization therapy: state of the art 2013. Eur Heart J 2013;34(19):1396–403.

18. Zhang J, Zhang Y, Zhou X, et al. QRS duration shortening predicts left ventricular reverse remodelling in patients with dilated cardiomyopathy after cardiac resynchronization therapy. Acta Cardiol 2015;70(3):307–13.

19. Sharma PS, Dandamudi G, Herweg B, et al. Permanent His-bundle pacing as an alternative to biventricular pacing for cardiac resynchronization therapy: a multicenter experience. Heart Rhythm 2018;15(3):413–20.

20. Shan P, Su L, Chen X, et al. Direct his-bundle pacing improved left ventricular function and remodelling in a biventricular pacing nonresponder. Can J Cardiol 2016;32(12):1577.e1-e4.

21. Barba-Pichardo R, Manovel Sanchez A, Fernandez-Gomez JM, et al. Ventricular resynchronization therapy by direct His-bundle pacing using an internal cardioverter defibrillator. Europace 2013;15(1):83–8.

22. Lustgarten DL, Crespo EM, Arkhipova-Jenkins I, et al. His-bundle pacing versus biventricular pacing in cardiac resynchronization therapy patients: a crossover design comparison. Heart Rhythm 2015;12(7):1548–57.

23. Ajijola OA, Upadhyay GA, Macias C, et al. Permanent his-bundle pacing for cardiac resynchronization therapy: initial feasibility study in lieu of left ventricular lead. Heart Rhythm 2017;14(9):1353–61.

24. Sharma PS, Ellison K, Patel HN, et al. Overcoming left bundle branch block by permanent His bundle pacing: evidence of longitudinal dissociation in the His via recordings from a permanent pacing lead. HeartRhythm Case Rep 2017;3(11):499–502.

25. Vijayaraman P, Dandamudi G. How to perform permanent his bundle pacing: tips and tricks. Pacing Clin Electrophysiol 2016;39(12):1298–304.

26. Vijayaraman P, Dandamudi G. Anatomical approach to permanent His bundle pacing: optimizing His bundle capture. J Electrocardiol 2016;49(5):649–57.

27. Sharma PS, Subzposh FA, Ellenbogen KA, et al. Permanent His-bundle pacing in patients with prosthetic cardiac valves. Heart Rhythm 2017;14(1):59–64.

28. Vijayaraman P, Dandamudi G, Worsnick S, et al. Acute his-bundle injury current during permanent his-bundle pacing predicts excellent pacing outcomes. Pacing Clin Electrophysiol 2015;38(5):540–6.

29. Zanon F, Svetlich C, Occhetta E, et al. Safety and performance of a system specifically designed for selective site pacing. Pacing Clin Electrophysiol 2011;34(3):339–47.

30. Kronborg MB, Mortensen PT, Poulsen SH, et al. His or para-His pacing preserves left ventricular function in atrioventricular block: a double-blind, randomized, crossover study. Europace 2014;16(8):1189–96.

31. Kronborg MB, Poulsen SH, Mortensen PT, et al. Left ventricular performance during para-His pacing in patients with high-grade atrioventricular block: an acute study. Europace 2012;14(6):841–6.

32. Su L, Xu L, Wu SJ, et al. Pacing and sensing optimization of permanent His-bundle pacing in cardiac resynchronization therapy/implantable cardioverter defibrillators patients: value of integrated bipolar configuration. Europace 2016;18(9):1399–405.

33. Saini A, Serafini N, Campbell S, et al. A novel, simple and accurate method for assessment of his bundle pacing morphology using near field and far field device electrograms. Heart Rhythm, in press.

Moving?

Make sure your subscription moves with you!

To notify us of your new address, find your **Clinics Account Number** (located on your mailing label above your name), and contact customer service at:

Email: journalscustomerservice-usa@elsevier.com

800-654-2452 (subscribers in the U.S. & Canada)
314-447-8871 (subscribers outside of the U.S. & Canada)

Fax number: 314-447-8029

Elsevier Health Sciences Division
Subscription Customer Service
3251 Riverport Lane
Maryland Heights, MO 63043

*To ensure uninterrupted delivery of your subscription, please notify us at least 4 weeks in advance of move.

ELSEVIER

Printed and bound by CPI Group (UK) Ltd, Croydon, CR0 4YY

13/10/2024

01773605-0001